My Journey Back to Oneness

by

Mark Allen Perkins

Artwork by Vince Sangmeister

Photography by Rose Boden

Printed in Victoria, Canada

National Library of Canada Cataloguing in Publication

Perkins, Mark
A journey back to oneness / written by Mark Perkins.
Includes bibliographical references.
ISBN 1-4120-0903-0
I. Title.

RZ999.P47 2003 615.8'9 C2003-904637-0

TRAFFORD

This book was published on-demand in cooperation with Trafford Publishing. On-demand publishing is a unique process and service of making a book available for retail sale to the public taking advantage of on-demand manufacturing and Internet marketing. **On-demand publishing** includes promotions, retail sales, manufacturing, order fulfilment, accounting and collecting royalties on behalf of the author.

Suite 6E, 2333 Government St., Victoria, B.C. V8T 4P4, CANADA
Phone 250-383-6864 Toll-free 1-888-232-4444 (Canada & US)
Fax 250-383-6804 E-mail sales@trafford.com
Web site www.trafford.com TRAFFORD PUBLISHING IS A DIVISION OF TRAFFORD HOLDINGS LTD.
Trafford Catalogue #03-1272 www.trafford.com/robots/03-1272.html

10 9 8 7 6 5 4

A Note of Gratitude

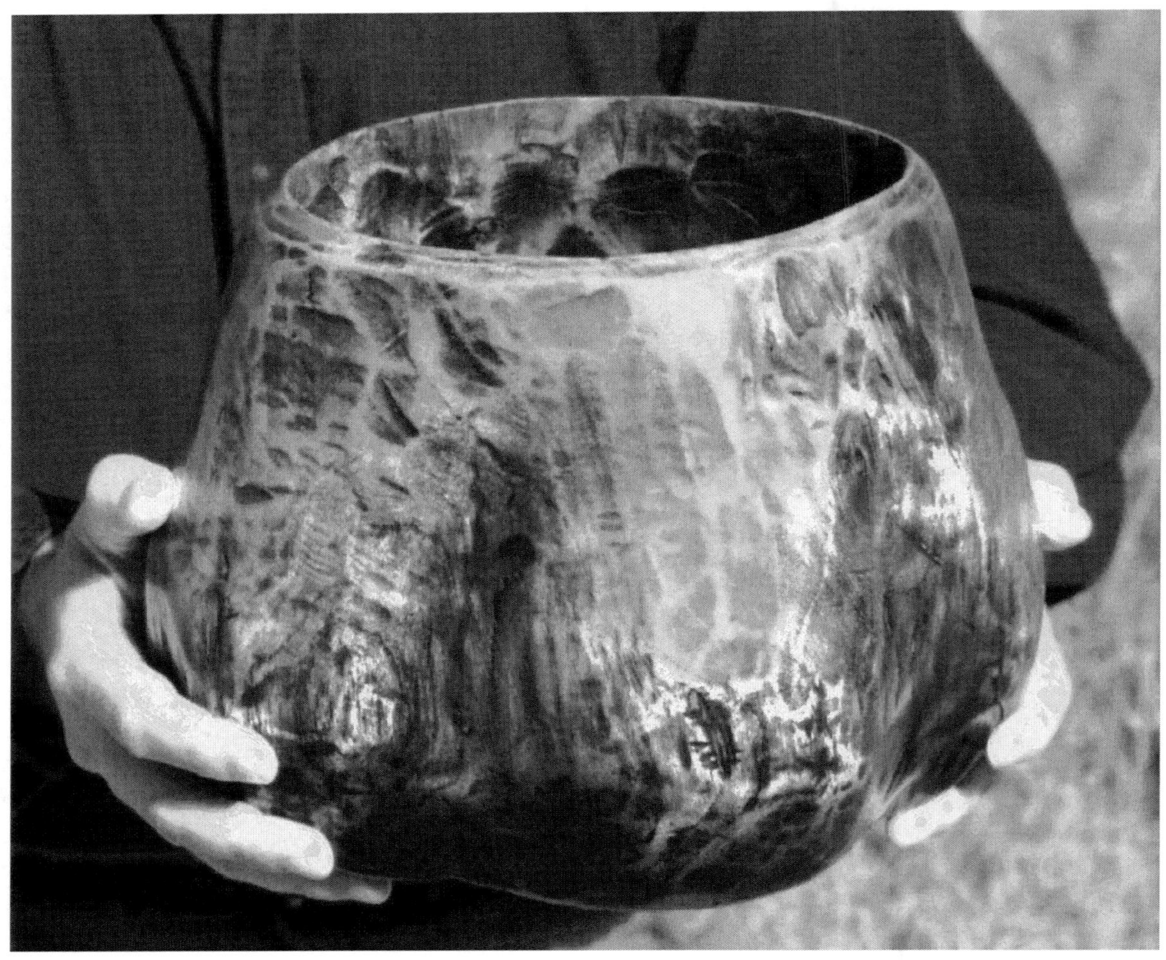

Photograph by Rose Boden

My "bowl of light" represents my mana or life force. To my readers, I offer you the gift of my energy through the words and pictures in this book.

Many people deserve my thanks for their support and help with this book. In particular, I would like to thank...

...my wife, Julie, for her support of my journey (all my love!),

...our children for their clear and uncluttered insight,

...my parents for their nurturing guidance,

...Hank Wesselman for stepping out,

...Cody and Robin for the inspiration,

...Rosie for her photographic talent,

..."Mister" Smith for his moral support,

...Vince for the inspired artwork (you did it!), and

...Laurie Keako'a' Grant. Sincere and heartfelt thanks go to her...the world and I owe her a debt of gratitude for her vision and her Ancient Rainbow Conscious Healing work.

Last, but certainly not least, I want to express my gratitude to the Divine Source.

Angel goes to work each day.

Takes care of her spouse and two kids.

Is a member of a sewing club.

Goes to church every Sunday.

Her life is full.

She is a success in her eyes.

She has just been diagnosed with cancer...

Why would a fair and loving God allow this to happen?

Why her?

Why your spouse?

Why me?

We spend a great deal of our lives, both awake and asleep, wondering about the great mysteries of our lives. Why am I here? What is the meaning of life? Why me? Is there a God?

Many of these questions are unanswerable at this point in our path of enlightenment as humans.

Many can be answered, if we allow ourselves to learn our lessons, accept the teaching the ailment is offering and...

Reconnect with the Divine Source!

Follow along on this journey back to Oneness.

Anyone who travels knows that there are numerous ways to get to a destination…a multitude of pathways, a myriad of methods…

The paths and methods chosen vary by person and circumstance…and are always subject to change at a moment's notice.

When I started down this book-writing path, I was headed in one direction, soon swept in another…influenced by my own experiences and the wisdom of others.

All the while, I was learning, growing and still moving towards the destination: Oneness!

At times, this trip has been exhilarating yet infuriating; pure joy and sheer agony, crystal clear and completely muddled – mostly because my analytical mind was trying to grasp Oneness concepts and methods and bridge between that realm and the one in which my physical body lives.

So, what you are about to read is a collection of my questions, analysis, insights and, at times, ramblings related to my personal journey back to Oneness…and the evidence that satisfied and completed my "logic circuit."

Many of the ideas that I have presented here are not new. Teachers and visionaries throughout time have offered these thoughts based on the premise that we:

- were all originally One
- began this existence with the full knowledge of that Oneness
- all need to get back to that Oneness.

In this book, I have attempted to document my connections between the different yet common ideas that have helped me in my journey back to Oneness.

I have found that it is difficult for some people to find and stay on their true path. I offer these insights because often times they attempt to take one teacher's ideas and use them as the only "map" on their path. I, too, had followed this type of focused approach early on. Through this book, I hope to show the reader the "maps" of many teachers – merged with my perceptions and analysis – in order to provide details for your own journey.

Look for my notes at the beginning of each chapter (in "boxed" text) that provide insight into how that topic fits into my journey thus far.

My hope is that after reading this, you will be encouraged to get out and "travel"...onward with the journey!

Shine!

– Mark Perkins
Boulder, CO – Spring 2004

Relax...

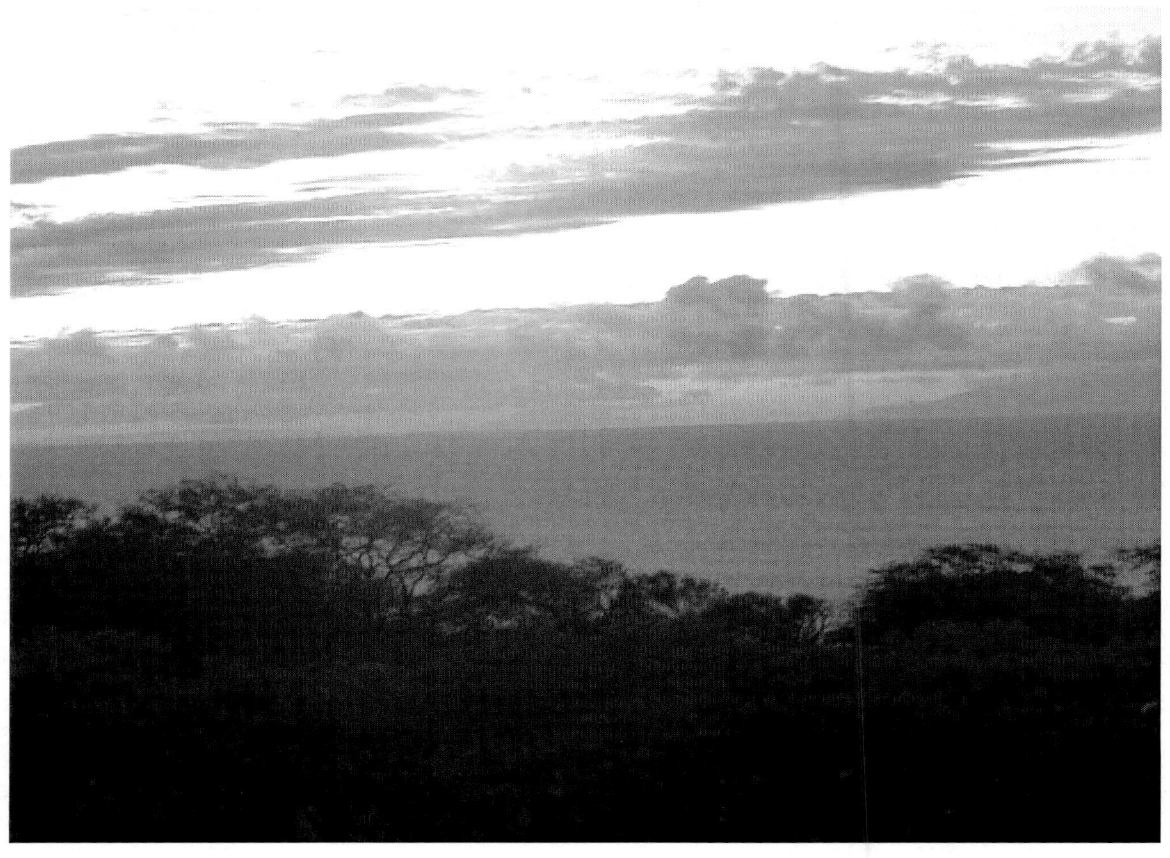

Photograph by Mark Perkins

View from the Kohala Coast of Hawaii

Come on a journey with me. It offers you the probability of experiencing healing on physical, mental and spiritual levels. This is a journey *back* to the place where we all started...a place of Oneness with the Divine Source. Are you interested?

As we begin this journey, I would like you to get comfortable. Take four deep breaths. In through the nose, holding your breath, then out through the mouth. I find that an inhale of five counts, holding for another five counts, then an exhale of five to ten counts, works nicely.

Allow your diaphragm and chest to expand fully. Feel the air filling your lungs. Concentrate on your breath. Clear your mind of your daily clutter. As thoughts arise, acknowledge them, thank them for offering the information and then let them go.

Take your first breath as most of us normally do, just with our lungs. On your second breath, feel yourself breathing with your whole body from the top of your head to the tip of your toes. On your third breath, fill beyond your skin...your house...your town...country...and beyond the Earth into space. On your fourth breath, feel the connection with the Divine!

Clear your mind...

In....Out...

In...Out...

In...Out...

In...Out...

Now that you are ready, I offer the following overview of what is to follow:

Our journey will begin in Chapter 1 with a refocusing of our perceptions of good and bad; us and them; and the other representation of duality that influences how we experience the world around us.

In Chapter 2, we will get a glimpse of the concepts behind Hawaiian mysticism and Shamanism – and establish the basic understanding of energy and reality as defined in these concepts.

A brief comparison of religious beliefs follows in Chapter 3 along with an exploration of prayer.

Chapters 4 and 5 explore the applications of the concepts addressed in the earlier chapters. We will examine how a Shamanic healer might go about enabling a client to heal and ground.

Throughout Chapters 1 to 5, I have attempted to impress upon you the ancient qualities and basic nature of the concepts discussed. In Chapter 6, I will attempt to make ties between these concepts and the origins of human beings.

Chapter 7, allows me to define how I see the future.

In the appendices, I recommend readings to further your knowledge, training to enhance the experiential nature of this type of work and descriptions of the artwork contained in these pages through the words of the artist.

Feel free to experience this work in the order that best suits your interests.

Chapter 1: Oneness Concepts

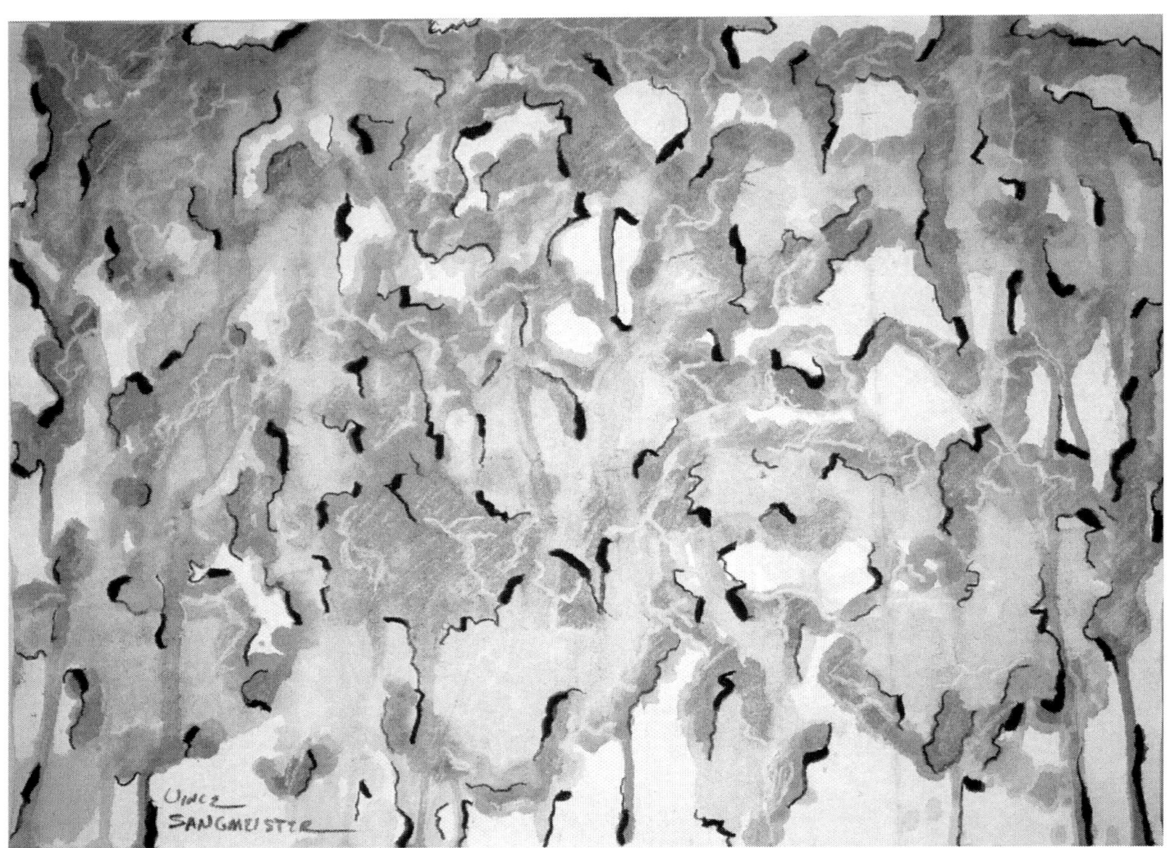

"Swift to Associate"

When a person starts on a journey, the images he or she sees are new, often muddled and difficult to distinguish. That person attempts to match his or her experiences to a rigid and learned understanding of the world. However, as you continue on the path, the hard and fast lines begin to "melt" – you begin to see the white light that is the background to all.

All things, material and spiritual, originate from one source and are related as if they were one family.

(From *Art of Peace* by Morihei Ueshiba O'Sensei © 1992 by John Stevens. Reprinted by arrangement with Shambhala Publications Inc., Boston – www.shambhala.com)

I thank my parents for placing me on a spiritual path. When I was growing up, my family put on our best clothes each Sunday and went to Sunday school and church. Due to various circumstances, I was blessed with the opportunity to experience different Christian denominations including Baptist, Methodist, Southern Baptist and Catholic. I was always taught about God and learned that the different denominations had varying practices – but they were all about the same thing: Jesus and God.

When I was about 13, we stopped going to church. At the time, my brothers and I thought this was great that we could stay home and watch cartoons! In pondering this decision, I have come to believe that my parents were giving me the opportunity to decide for myself what I believed in, so that I could create my own spiritual path.

This chapter represents what I have come to realize about Oneness principles through my:

- Early church experiences
- Study and practice of Aikido (a Japanese "martial art")
- Research about Shamanism and numerous religions (more on this in Chapters 2 and 3)

Questions answered for me in this chapter include:

- What are the key Oneness concepts?
- Why is he angry?

“Good” and “Bad”

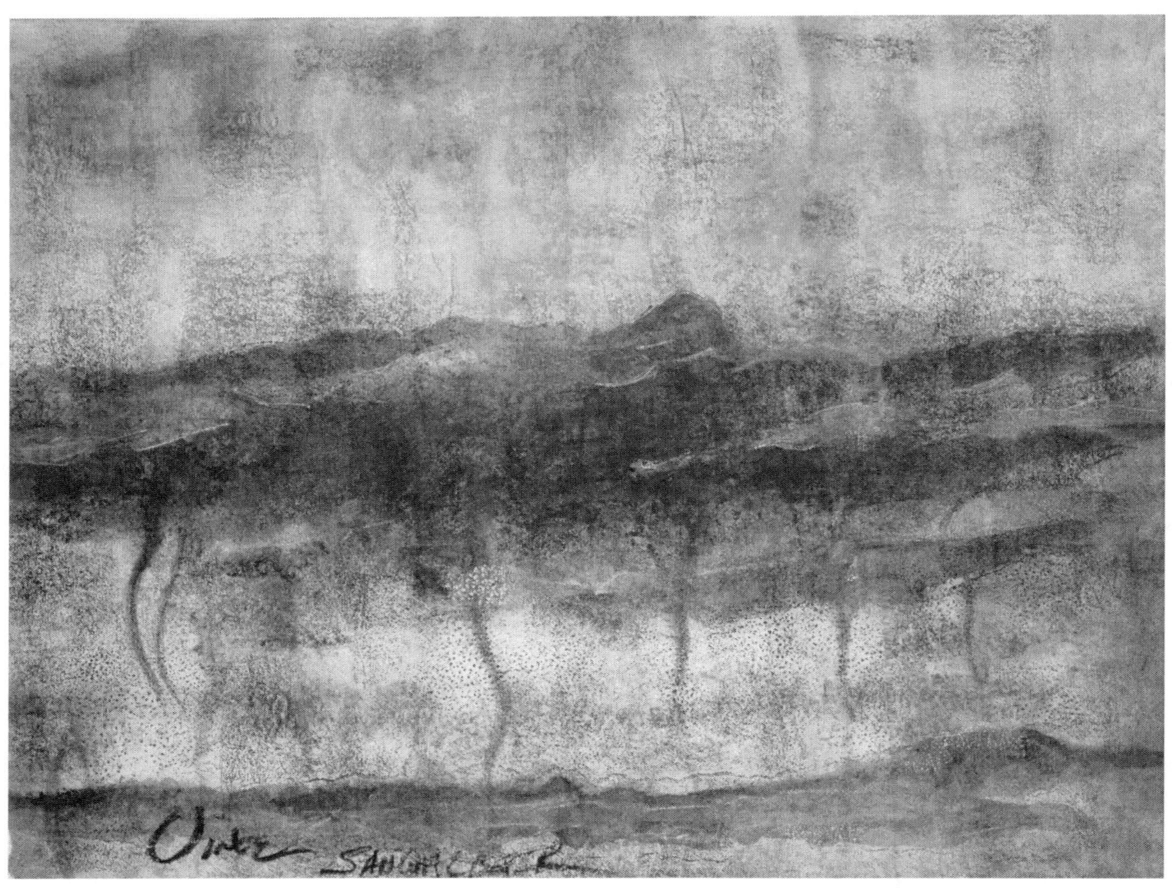

“CD1 Cut1”

A storm is approaching. You know that soon the wind will blow and the rain will pour, but, after a “bad” storm, the clear, cool, “good” air will fill your lungs. The fish will come...new and wonderful discoveries await. You will experience many storms...however, they are all good...

The goal of Oneness is to reconnect you with God, YHWH, Divine Source, Great Spirit – or the name that you use to describe the Universal Oneness that is the source of all – and to help you get back in touch with that Spirit. I say "back" because we are all born with that strong Oneness connection. We know this when we are children. Some very lucky people carry this knowledge with them throughout their whole life. However, many of us are "societized" out of it and live our lives in "duality" – right/wrong, good/bad, us/them.

The objective is for you to rediscover the grand plan for your life and to realize that you are not just out there flailing on your own. The Bible, in John 15:5, quotes Jesus as saying, "I am the vine and you are the branches." This is a very powerful statement addressing the concept of Oneness. We are all part of the plant or complete entity. We cannot separate ourselves from the rest of the plant without dying. When we acknowledge our Oneness, we move from simply surviving (subsisting in a day-to-day existence of consuming nutrients, exhaling carbon dioxide and watching the world go by) to truly living.

There are many ways to achieve Oneness, through many different methods – for example: meditation, Shamanic journeying, healing modalities, practices of organized religions, etc.

The concepts and methods you will read about in this book are in no way a religion in the formal, accepted definition, although the ideas are addressed throughout various religions. I offer them as enhancements to your existing practices, whatever they may be.

Returning to Oneness with the Divine Source will allow you to grow and flourish with the knowledge that you are not alone. As your Oneness connection grows, you will consistently begin to recognize that the Divine Source is in all, both the "good" and the "bad."

So, let us start by looking at some of the basic Oneness concepts. The first concept is "Good" and "Bad."

In the words of Heraclitus, a Greek philosopher from the 6th-century B.C., "To God, all things are beautiful, good and right. Men, on the other hand, deem some things right and others wrong."

"Good" and "bad" are misnomers. **All situations are good and are gifts from the Divine Source to help us to grow**. Sometimes it is very difficult to fathom the good that is contained in horrible acts, but that is not for you or me to decide. Human nature seems to dictate that we personalize everything that happens in the world. This is probably the by-product of our ability to receive news and communications from next door or the other side of world equally quick. This personalization causes someone to feel directly affected by a situation that is not part of his or her path or lessons to learn.

Many people go through life after the death of a love one wondering, "Why me?" They feel that they were and still are being punished. I offer that it is highly possible that the death of a loved one was part of the loved one's path. It was part of his or her lesson to be learned...not yours. We need to have compassion for situations in the world where there is suffering and pain but we also need to understand that the situation may not have anything to do with us personally. If you look closely, you can learn to distinguish between when it is your lesson to be learned and another's chance to learn. When you are in a situation, meditate or "do a gut check" or open yourself to the energy of the Divine. If you do, you will receive an answer as to whether you have a part in what is happening. Many times the answer is not a verbal yes or no. It might be a bird singing that makes you feel happy or some other outside stimulus that gives you pleasure. I read these signs as an indicator that, however unpleasant the situation may be, it is not mine. Similarly, when you get your answer and still feel "connected" to the situation, there is something in the situation that is there to support your path and learning. It is now up to you to determine what the lesson is. We will discuss some ways to help you find this knowledge later in the book.

I liken attempts to understand the plans of the Divine Source to a child trying to understand why his parent would take him to the "Doctor" for immunizations. There, a person in a white coat plunges a needle into the child's leg then smiles and says, "There, all better." In the moment of pain, the child is definitely not able to realize the long-term benefit.

We are but children when it comes to understanding actions done at the vibrational level of the Divine Source.

I have truly come to believe that we are all one with each other and the Divine Source! A main component of this concept is the knowledge that your thoughts, actions, feelings, motivations and emotions throughout every moment of your life are being directed, encouraged and fostered by the Divine Source. As such, you need to be consciously aware of what energies you are offering to your environment.

Are you putting out positive thoughts?

Have you witnessed something that one might consider to be appalling and you know that there must be something behind the incident that is part of a greater plan, whether you can comprehend the plan or not?

Have you ever noticed that when you hold the thought that things can never go right, they do not?

We will talk further about co-creation later in this book, but as a preview consider this: the Divine Source is constantly providing energy to us that is acted upon by our thoughts, feelings and emotions. If we are thinking thoughts that encourage harmony; harmony manifests. If we are feeling fear; fear pervades. We are constantly offered the energy to change our environment. It is up to us to decide.

Take September 11th, 2001 for example. Many, many people died tragically during that event. It was and is still difficult to grasp what possible good could become of an action so devastating. However, shortly afterwards, I observed several media reports that sales of the Koran had risen sharply. People, while they may have not believed in the actions taken by the individuals responsible for the incident, wanted to learn more about Islam. They wanted to understand the Islamic faith better.

In addition, during this incident and its aftermath, did you notice how New York, the United States and the World came together?

Did you see miracles and heroism?

All of these "good" things were manifesting in the most "horrid" of situations.

These situations are what my ohana (family) calls "blessons"[1] – a blessing and a lesson all rolled into one!

Seeing the "blessons" in the resulting acts of heroism and the increased sales of the Koran can go a long way towards understanding that we are all one – and that the actions of the few do not represent the ideas of the many. After reading the Koran, many people found that the ideas expressed in it are not much different from the beliefs of their own (and other) religions or practices.

The reason it may be hard to see these similarities can partly be attributed to the cultural "brush strokes" that are painted on top of religious beliefs. Things like: you cannot eat fish on Friday, or do not eat any pork, or you may not drink fermentation of the wheat or vine. Additionally, political "brush strokes" like "allies" or "axis of evil" also cause us not to see common themes like Love your Neighbor, Respect Nature, Be Thankful, etc.

Regardless of these cultural and political "brush strokes," the underlying idea is the same: There is one true God or Source, who loves and cares for all...and we are all part of that Divine Energy!

---

1 A special "Thank You" to Rhonda.

You get Back what You put Out

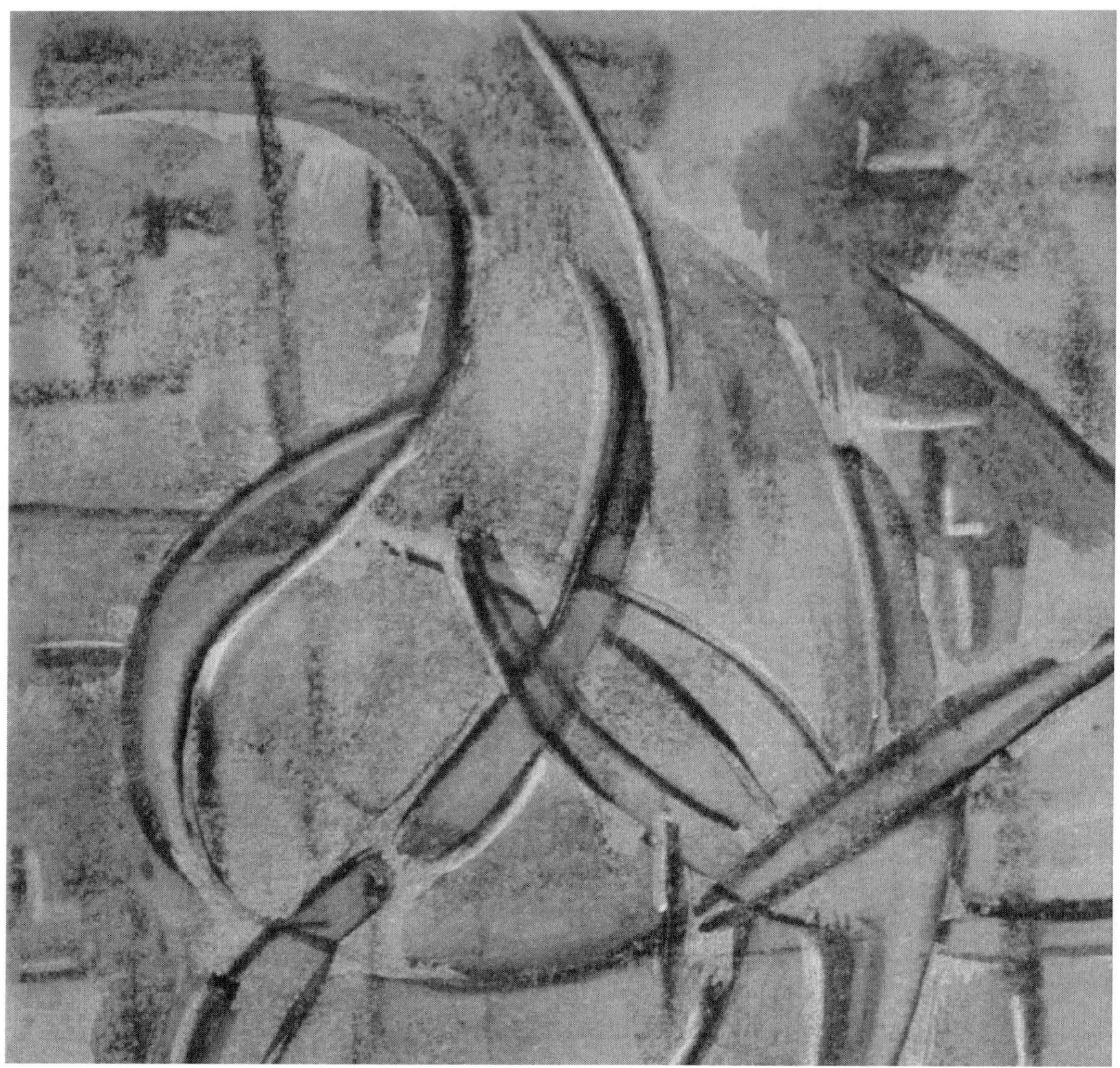

"Metropolitan Vortices" (detail)

Especially in an urban center, there is a constant stream of energy that we, sometimes unconsciously, release into our environment, like vortices spiraling and mingling together to co-create our reality. Are you helping to create the optimal environment?

The energy that you radiate is what appears in the world. The notion that "you get back what you put out" is another key Oneness concept. To illustrate this point, I want you to do the following exercise...

Recall a positive thought or situation. It could be a childhood memory, the birth of a child, your wedding, or whatever creates a pleasant emotion – one that really affirms the Divine in all things. Think about that situation and pay attention. Experience how simply remembering the situation changes your body. Things in your environment are brighter and prettier. Scents and sounds are stronger and more vibrant. Foods taste better. You smile.

How do you feel?

Now I would like you to remember something that is unpleasant. Let us start simple and not call upon memories that are extreme. Try this: recall the smell of garbage or the stench from a dumpster. Notice how you react when you experience these smells. You frown. You might cringe. You may think about walking on the other side of the street just to avoid the situation.

Now how do you feel?

Have you ever noticed that, like the old songs says, "When you're smiling, the whole world smiles with you?"[2]

The opposite is also true.

This was a very simple example of your thoughts, feelings and emotions causing physical manifestations even when the actual physical stimulus is not present. When you are positive, you smile. When you are negative, you pull back. Your actions and reactions are also sent out into the world. When you think something positive, you might say "hello" to the next person that you meet and pass on some of your positive energy – to another person and to the world. By doing a simple act like this, you may have shown someone else the door to allow them to smile and propagate the feeling further. Others are guaranteed to feel this.

---

2 "When You're Smiling, the Whole World Smiles with You" – words and music by Mark Fisher, Joe Goodwin and Larry Shay, 1928.

Sometimes this often appears to fail. Someone may be so very engrossed in his or her own drama that your positive energy is overlooked by the conscious mind. However, the unconscious "sees" and a reaction occurs. Because the unconscious can see, it holds the positive thought, feeling or emotion that you are transmitting in order to reinforce that person's unconscious with constructive thoughts, feelings and emotions.

The lesson here? Put out "positive" – and do not be drawn in by the negative thoughts, feelings and emotions that someone else may be transmitting.

Seeing from the Other's Eyes

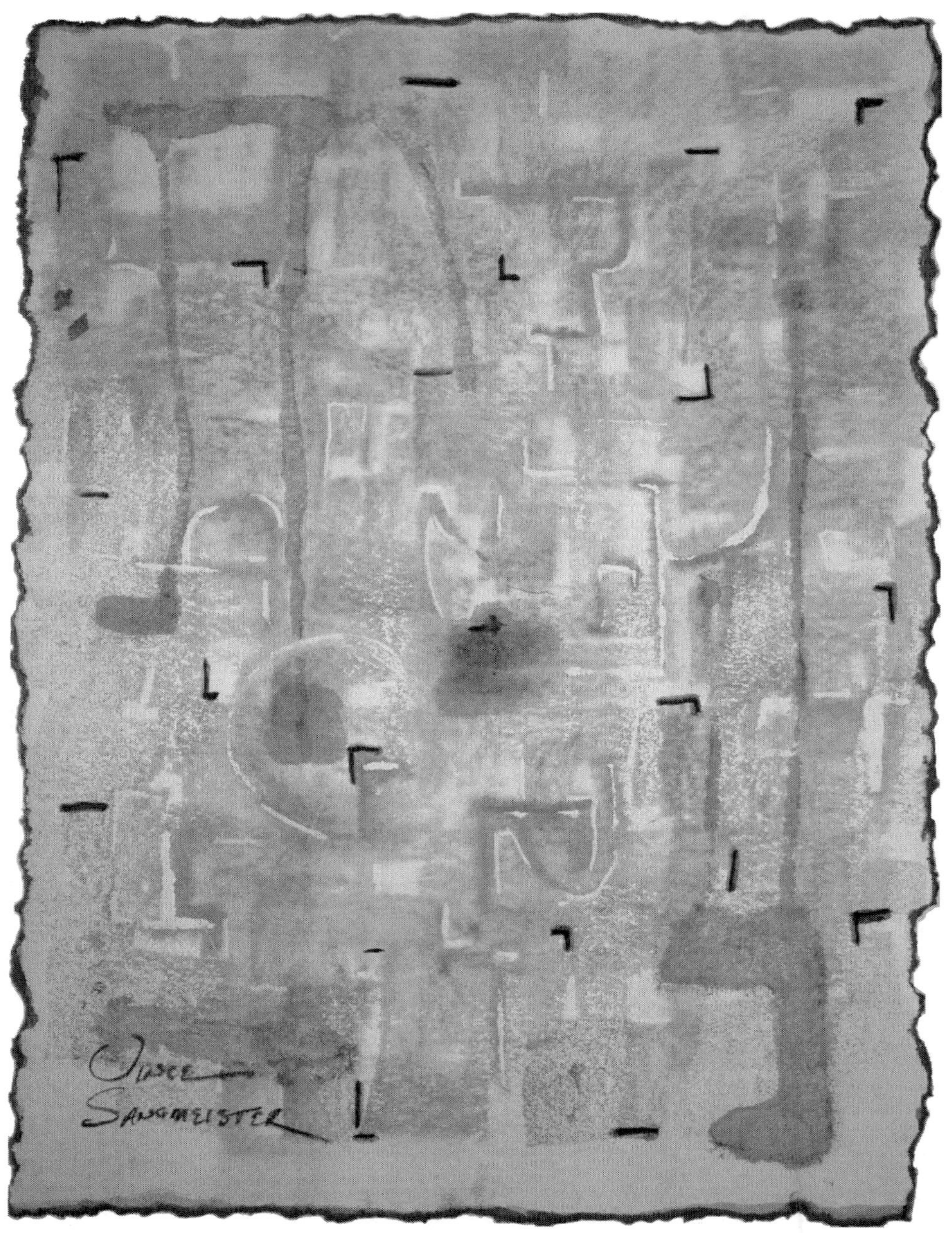

"Filtered and Refocused"

Seeing from someone else's eyes is like using someone else's glasses. Things look filtered and blurry until you can adjust your focus.

My path has been and continues to be an adventure. It has included a tour of duty in the U.S. Marine Corps where I learned both sides of life: taking and preserving. We were trained dutifully in killing the enemy before he could kill us. I was then taught to gather intelligence information that could be used to save lives. I continued with this job as a civilian with the Department of Defense. I was trying to work within the system in an attempt to make it less of a war machine and more of a benefit to all humanity.

I do not know if I succeeded, but I know that my teammates and I did all we could to keep the world safe. During this time, as a logical continuation of my path, I began to study Aikido. This Japanese "martial art" was the catalyst that propelled me along my spiritual journey.

The principles that form the foundation of Aikido really resonated with me. It was not until several years later that I realized that they were my first introduction to Oneness concepts. I would like to share these Aikido principles with you now.

Morihei Ueshiba O'Sensei invented Aikido in the early 20th century. The primary purpose of Aikido is to unite the world. This is accomplished not by forcing everyone to see things a certain way, but by:

- allowing individuals to maintain their uniqueness, and
- seeing their point of view not as foreign, but as a part of the whole.

The aim of Aikido is compassion expressed through the spirit of budo. Budo has many definitions depending on your path. Many people translate budo as the "martial way" or the "way of war." In Aikido, budo is defined in its most ancient and purest form as the "way of stopping the spear" or "path of peace."

To break down the essence of Aikido further, the word "aikido" can be translated as follows:

Ai – love

Ki – the universal life force

Do – way or path

Therefore, Aikido can be translated as the "way of love through the universal life force." As explained by Aikido World Headquarters,[3] Aikido teaches that budo combined with the spirit of heaven and earth in your heart, can fulfill your life's destiny with unconditional love for everything. Aikido is the path of forgiveness and enlightenment. At the heart of Aikido is the Eastern concept of Ki – the universal creative principle and universal life force. This energy is also known as Chi in China, Prana in India and Mana is Polynesia. Aikido seeks to unite universal Ki (Divine Source Energy) with the Ki (life force or breath) found within each person.

Aikido is based on the movements found in nature. These are efficient, rational and soft, while the center is immovable, firm and stable. The principle of a firm center is universally consistent. Many cultures speak of centering and "finding one's center" as the basis for enlightenment. The culmination of Aikido is expressed by aligning one's center or Ki with the center expressed throughout nature.

There is a wonderful theory in Aikido that reinforces this principle. In a situation where an antagonist "pushes" you, what is your first reaction? Push back? Run away? Hide?

For many, the first reaction is to push back. When you push back, you have "received" the thoughts, feelings and emotions of fear and anger that were transmitted to you by the antagonist and you have placed yourself on that level. You are now transmitting fear and anger by pushing back.

One of the teachings of Aikido is to see the situation from the antagonists' point of view. Why are the antagonists angry? How did they get into this situation? Are they having a bad day? Was there a recent traumatic situation? Death in the family? Sickness? What has upset them to such a degree that you are perceived as a threat and they need to be afraid and/or take action? To them, did you do something offensive?

If you try to put yourself in the antagonists' shoes and see things from their point of view, it might help you to understand why the negative actions were taken. Seeing it from their viewpoint will help you understand the thoughts, feelings and emotions under which they are operating. Hopefully, this knowledge will allow you to understand and redirect their actions so that all parties are safe and the situation is diffused without violence. If you add the movements of Aikido into this scenario, they would allow situations to be neutralized – and show aggressors that their current path is not beneficial to the overall harmony of the universe.

---

3 For additional information, see http://www.aikikai.or.jp

Like many other spiritually conscious individuals, you may have a meditation regimen that you follow. When a thought comes up during meditation, I have been taught to acknowledge the thought and let it go. Likewise, in order to redirect negative energy, identify why the person was acting in a violent manner then let the situation blend with your positive thoughts, feelings and emotions while maintaining your stable, focused center. This allows the antagonist the opportunity to allow his or her anger to dissipate and stop the proliferation of violence.

We, as keepers of this Earth, need to be better in understanding the people that do not think, act or feel like us. We need to embrace them as equals so that we may understand their points of view and they, ours. No one wins in war. From a point of view based on the teachings of Aikido, the focus is harnessing the power of the attacker's anger and fear, and then redirecting that power so that you **and** the attacker are not harmed. You move in such a way as to see from the attacker's point of view. You evaluate the motives from a safe position for both entities involved. Decisions are made with a mutual understanding of the perceptions of everyone concerned.

A portal is available.

Open that door to the person and demonstrate that there are other ways to deal with the situation and that the world is not the enemy. The world is part of him or her – and he or she are a part of it.

We are all One.

The previous ideas and examples lead us back to Oneness and the beautiful Divine Source Energy that is in everything. Divine Source Energy is even with the person who is angry. Seeing the essence of the Divine Source in all, allows everyone to learn the lessons offered. By learning our lessons, we can guide each other back into our original higher vibrational realm.

In this higher realm, Oneness helps us heal our thoughts, feelings, emotions and, ultimately, our souls. When we acknowledge that there are lessons to be learned, (e.g. compassion, patience, common courtesy, etc.) and we accept those lessons, we have healed an aspect of ourselves.

The study of Aikido has been integral in my understanding of my "dark side." The "dark side" has been defined as the part of an entity that delivers ego-driven reactions to situations. This part pushes back when pushed. This part sees things as separate, dark and light, good and bad. Aikido has shown, and is showing me, that I must "see from the other's eyes" in order to achieve true Oneness and heal my dark side.

Not long ago, I was discussing the concept of war with my elder kumu or teacher. I was trying to understand what it would take to stop war forever. Kumu said that as some of us grow and begin to understand that war does not solve problems, there are "younger" souls waiting to take up arms and be the "warriors." This wisdom reminded me of the words of the chief in the book *Hanta Yo,*[4] who wondered if he had grown to such an age that he no longer had the heart for war. The chief also acknowledged that the young braves were ready, willing and able to take his place in war and in guiding the tribe.

I see Aikido as the path for the older warrior, the one who sees that killing another is killing a part of him or her. The path allows the elder to continue to lead the tribe through experience and wisdom. This same path is available for the young warriors who have the desire and skill to protect their people. If they manifest this protection through a respect for <u>all</u> life, not just the lives of their own people, perhaps the following generations of warriors will not know war.

In Aikido, there is not a winner or loser…just life.

---

4 *Hanta Yo* by Ruth Beebe Hill, published by Doubleday & Company, Inc., ISBN: 0-385-13554-8.

Chapter 2: Shamanism

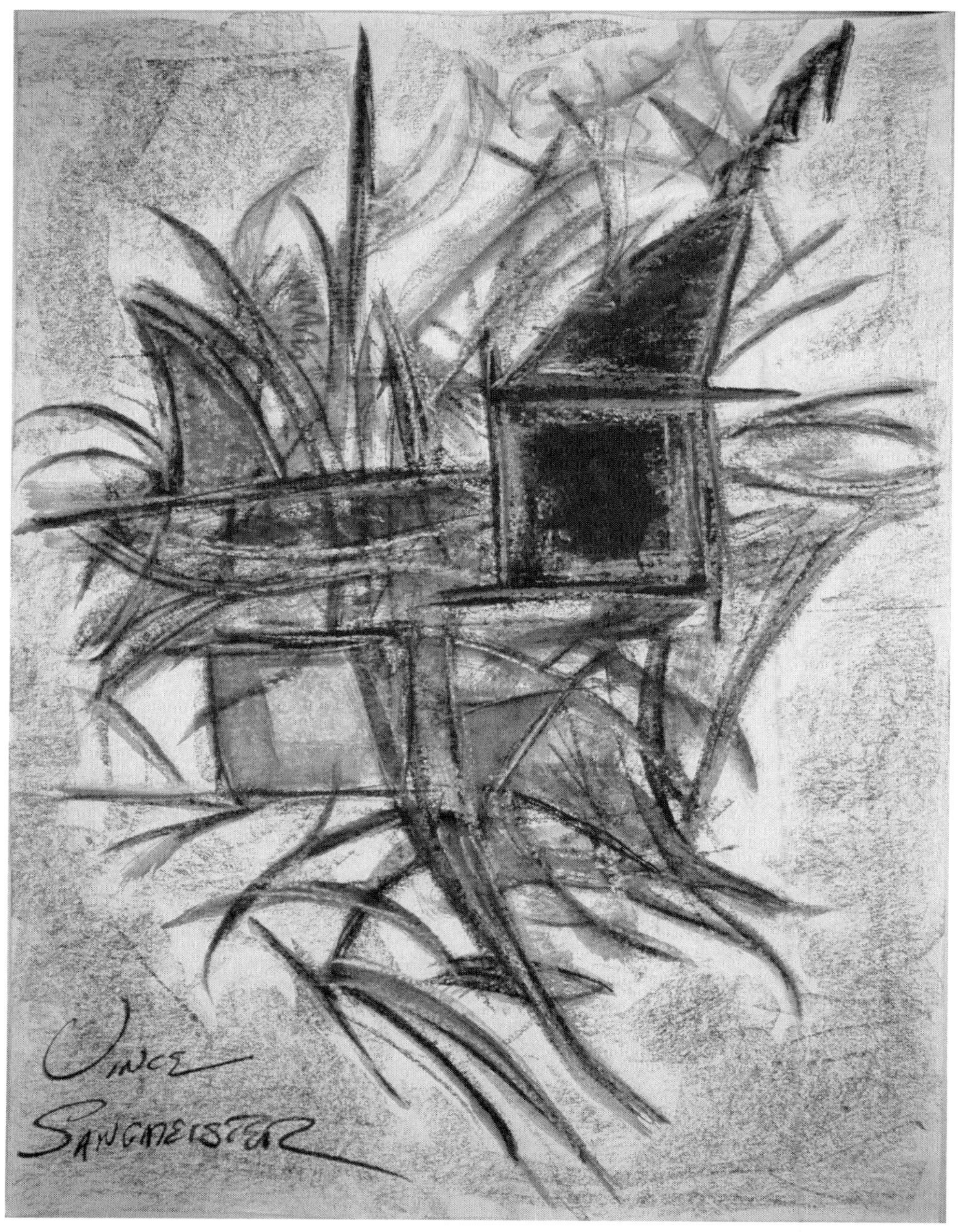

"Lucid Dream II"

There is a "jungle" that is our everyday life. It clouds the perception of non-ordinary reality and the tunnel that leads one there.

My first introduction to any kind of "healing" (other than Western medicine) was in 1996 when my wife experienced a Reiki session in Maryland, where we were living at the time. Reiki, an ancient form of hands-on healing, helped her through a major life transition and started her on a Spiritual path. I was intrigued by her descriptions of how good she felt...I wanted to investigate Reiki more and possibly even learn it, so that I could help my wife have those feelings on a regular basis.

It was not until we moved West that I had that opportunity. I took a Reiki class taught by Laurie Grant in Boulder, CO. From the moment that class started, Laurie and I were in sync. We had a connection that made it very easy for me to understand and absorb the information.

When Laurie moved on to "re-discover" Ancient Rainbow Conscious Healing, I continued to study with her for a couple of years.

During those years, the old "intelligence analyst" in me (the one who spent 15-years analyzing information and studying language / cultures for the Department of Defense) was very curious about the origins of Hawaiian healing and Spiritual practices. Therefore, I did what I knew how to do best: research. That is when I found Shamanism.

During my research, I found the teachings of many experts in this field. I have had the pleasure to study under Dr. Hank Wesselman, Sandra Ingerman, Gregg Braden, Barbara Marx Hubbard and Dan Millman, in addition to Laurie Grant. Their teachings (referenced in Appendix A) have furthered my journey on this path to Oneness – and are recommended reading for you too!

Questions answered for me in this chapter include:

- What is Shamanism?
- How does a Shaman view the world?
- How does the Shaman facilitate healing?

Hawaiian Mysticism

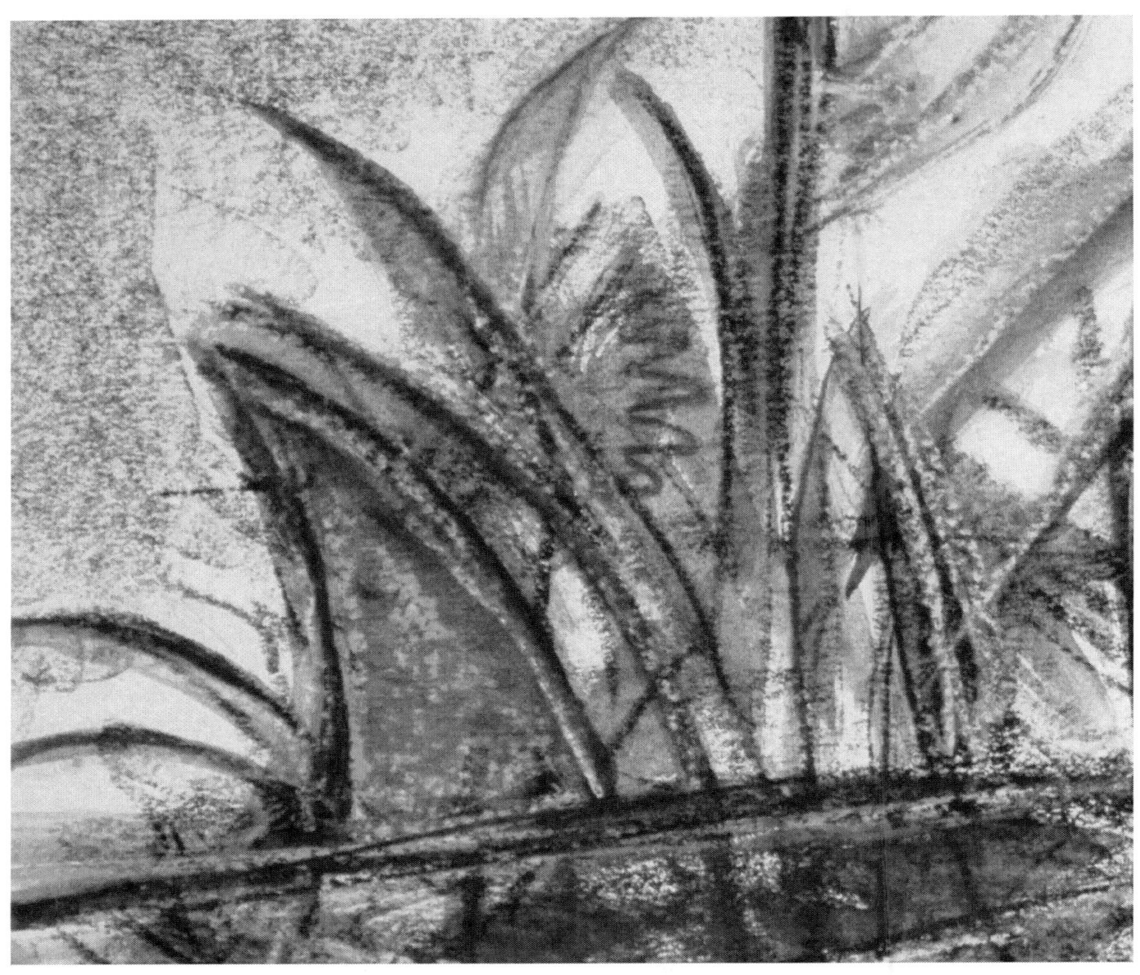

"Lucid Dream II" (detail)

Sometime the jungle is very close and oppressive...Tough to see the forest...

My experiences with Oneness are rooted in the teachings of the Kahuna Shamans of Hawaii. However, this lineage of healing through Oneness is more ancient than Hawaii and we will discuss the antiquity of this ancestry further in a later chapter.

In looking at religions throughout the world, you will find that many belief systems recognize that we are all part of the Divine Source. However, few religions truly reinforce this knowledge as part of its believer's daily lives. The concept of Oneness with the Divine was and is, to some extent, an integral part of the culture and religious practices of the ancient Polynesians.

Many belief systems identify Oneness with a master or leader. The ancient Hawaiians believed that everyone and everything were a representation of the Divine and, as such, were treated as one would treat the Divine.

There are several Hawaiian myths concerning Oneness. While many of the details of the ancient wisdom are shrouded in secrecy and cultural dogma, the main theme is realizing that you are not, and have never been, separate from the Divine Source.

One of the aspects of this key theme is the release of blockages. A blockage is a "piece of baggage" or "stone" that you are carrying that keeps you from fully healing. In *VisionSeeker: Shared Wisdom from the Place of Refuge*[5] and in *Tales from the Night Rainbow*,[6] the authors relate an ancient Hawaiian healing tradition of the accumulation of "stones" in a bowl that holds our life force energy. The stones represent instances when you have been jealous, judgmental, uncaring, cruel – in general, negative. The more stones you have, the less room there is for the light or life force. How does one get rid of these stones? Simply turn the bowl over and pour them out! This symbolic dumping of our old ways of thinking, issues, wrongdoings, etc. removes the blockages to healing.

In order to achieve a more complete healing, one must accept the "blesson" (a blessing and a lesson!) that they need to learn and dump out the blockages that are holding them back from complete healing. An example of this can be found in patients who survived cancer and felt it was the best thing that ever happened to them. They appreciate life more, see the beauty of the world clearer and live life to the fullest. Many of us have also seen this type of reaction with heart attack victims. Survivors re-discover life as a gift to be cherished. They are able to learn their lessons, remove the blockage of being a "victim" and heal.

---

5 *VisionSeeker: Shared Wisdom from the Place of Refuge* by Dr. Hank Wesselman, published by Hay House, ISBN: 1-56170-753-8.

6 *Tales from the Night Rainbow* by Koko Willis and Pali Jae Lee, published by Night Rainbow Publishing Company, ISBN: 0-9628030-0-6.

Just as a lesson can be the foundation for a developing illness, the normally unconscious perception that being "sick" is to our benefit can be a powerful thought form. So powerful in fact, that it can lead to actual physical illness. I, myself, have had instances where I believed that my desire not to do something has led to injury or illness. If we look closely, we all do or have done this at one time or another.

When we...

- acknowledge that there are lessons to be learned,
- accept our lessons,
- keep our bowls of light stone-free,
- realize that everything is an aspect of the Divine Source, and
- "co-create" by using the energy offered by the Divine Source...

...then we have a formula that provides the basis for a lifelong spiritual path!

We also achieve a state that leads to complete healing on all aspects of our past, present and future lives.

As we discussed earlier, my study of Oneness is based on the beliefs of ancient Polynesia, specifically Hawaii. The priestly leaders that facilitated these beliefs were the Kahuna.

The Kahuna can be classified as the Shamans of Hawaii. As with other Shamans throughout the world, the Kahuna were the keepers of the wisdom and spirituality of their race. They were respected as healers and visionaries that would shepard their people through life and help guide them on the path to spiritual enlightenment.

A Kahuna is an expert. There were and still are, Kahuna for navigation, fishing, building, healing, woodworking, war and just about anything else at which you can imagine a person being an expert. Kahuna are the seers.

They are intimately familiar with their chosen trade. Some examples: hunter Kahuna would find their prey by "connecting" with the animal and asking the quarry's help in the survival of the Kahuna's people. Navigator Kahuna spent years watching the stars, currents, weather – and learned shipbuilding techniques in order to give the greatest probability of a successful open-ocean journey. They also merged with the atmosphere prior to the journey to ask assistance.

Much of the direct knowledge of how Kahuna accomplished their connection with nature and the spirit worlds has been lost. However, one potential link does still exist: Shamanism.

The Shaman

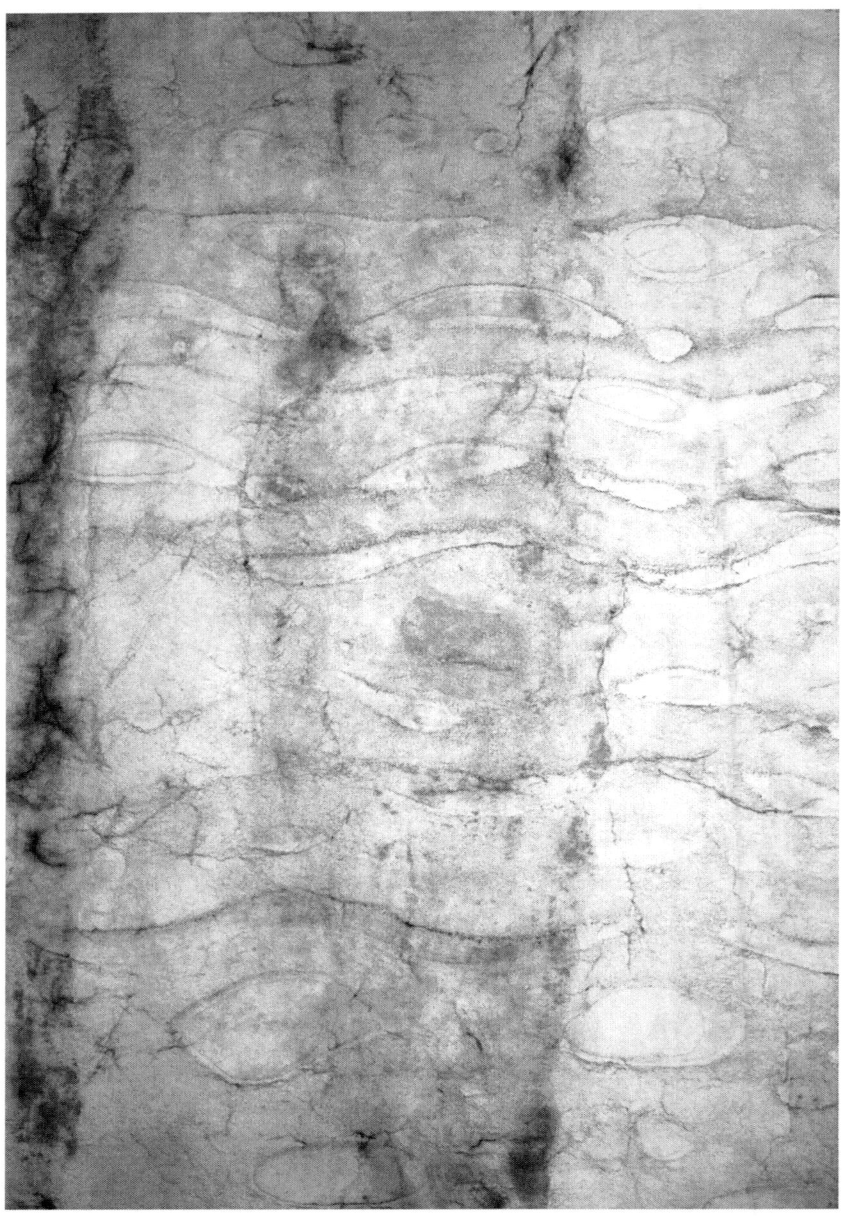

"CD1 Cut1" (bleed through image on back, detail)

Vince, the artist, was not aware that this image existed. We discovered it while photographing the images. I see the outline of a vaguely human form and at the top, middle of the image; I see the eyes, nose and mouth of a helping spirit that I have seen in non-ordinary reality.

Shamanistic practices have been observed in all cultures, in every era. Shamans utilize a close relationship with nature to facilitate their abilities of prophecy and healing. Like in the Hawaiian belief system, Shamans also understand that the root of ailment is not bacteria or viruses, but a physical, spiritual, psychological imbalance and/or lesson to be learned.

Modern medicine has also begun to realize this possibility. Dr. Marilyn Schlitz, PhD, describes multiple personality cases in which there were "...people who have in one personality a particular kind of condition – for example, they may be diabetic, needing a high level of insulin – while in another personality, they seem to need less insulin, or none at all. One personality may be allergic to cats; the other is not. There is more and more evidence that there is something about this plasticity of the body and its relationship to the mind and to consciousness that has yet to be accommodated within the conventional medical model."[7]

Deepak Chopra also describes this type of phenomenon in his book *Quantum Healing*.[8]

There are many different practices employed by Shamans. The work of Michael Harner[9] has centered on finding the common threads amongst the varying Shamanic practices. These common themes include the concepts of ordinary and non-ordinary reality and three worlds.

As taught in the workshops of Michael Harner[10] and Dr. Hank Wesselman,[11] ordinary reality is the world we live in. It is the physical reality of our five senses. It is the world that we describe through our chemistry and physics, the conscious mind and faith. In this reality, there is separateness: a beginning and an end; a cause and an effect.

---

7 From a speech by Marilyn Schlitz, PhD at the June 1998 Comprehensive Cancer Care Conference which was jointly sponsored by The Center For Mind-Body Medicine, James S. Gordon, MD, Director, National Institutes of Health's (NIH) Office of Alternative Medicine (OAM) and the University of Texas-Houston Health Science Center Medical School of Nursing.

8 *Quantum Healing: Exploring the Frontiers of Mind Body Medicine* by Deepak Chopra, published by Bantam Books, ISBN 0553348698.

9 Michael Harner outlines his research into the common teachings of Shamans throughout the world in *The Way of the Shaman*, published by Harper San Francisco, ISBN 0062503731.

10 Further information on training offered by Harner's Foundation for Shamanic Studies can be found at http://www.Shamanism.org.

11 See http://www.sharedwisdom.com for Dr. Wesselman's training schedule.

Non-ordinary reality is the world of spirit. It is the world of dreams, spirits and intuition. It is where all things are conscious. It is the place of "no time" where the past, present and future all exist and are accessible. It is the place where thoughts, feelings and emotions create our physical reality and is the spirit mirror of our ordinary reality. In this place, all is connected and related. It is a place of symbolism. The Shaman "journeys" to non-ordinary reality to access the information contained therein. He then uses this data to help facilitate healing in ordinary reality.

Non-ordinary reality is commonly viewed as three distinct areas or worlds: lower, middle and upper.

The lower world is the realm of animal spirits, nature, earth energies, etc. In the lower world, one can ground energies and influence the state of the physical body. In journeys to this world, the Shaman can find information to help with survival, sexual and balance issues. It is the place where you can find "safety." It is the realm of fairies, brownies, sprites, animal helpers, elves and devas. Here, the hunting Shaman would connect with the spirit of his prey and ask permission to take the animal's life, honor it and thank it for its gifts.

The middle world is the domain of compassion. It is the place of rest for the soul. In the middle world, the Shaman connects with the spirits of departed loved ones, souls, beings, spirits and guides. It is where the lono or mind influences thoughts, feelings and emotions and directs the ku or physical. When a Shaman does distance healing,[12] the middle world is the starting point. It is also the location of each person's private healing garden, a place we can create ourselves and visit often.[13]

The upper world is the home of one's aumakua or over-soul. This world is the mother of intuition and influencer of the mental functions. It is the guide of our actions that has the benefit of knowing all things. It does not, however, speak in plain language. It speaks in metaphor and symbols that the Shaman must interpret and place in context in order to use the information. This is where the Shaman travels to past and future realms to gain knowledge.

Although viewed as distinct worlds, these areas often blend and allow one to experience a balance of information supplied by helpers in each world.

---

12 Distance healing is when the healer provides energy to someone or something at a distance. This distance can be as close as the next room or as far as across the world.

13 *The Journey to the Sacred Garden: A Guide to Traveling in the Spiritual Realms* by Dr. Hank Wesselman, published by Hay House, Inc., ISBN 1401901115, provides a detailed description of a healing garden and how to create it.

Access to this non-ordinary realm is activated by:

Percussive beat	Drum, rattle, didgeridoo, singing bowl, chanting, etc.
Breath work	Controlled, conscious breathing that will build up the Shaman's supply of mana or energy.
Bribery	Promising the ku a physically pleasurable experience like food, music, sex, etc.
Pain	Physical pain, fasting, etc. as demonstrated through numerous Native American and other indigenous cultures' rituals.
Drugs	Hallucinogenic substances used by indigenous cultures to remove the veil of ordinary reality including peyote, mescal, mushrooms, etc.

The belief system of the Hawaiians is closely aligned with the Shamanistic view of the world. In Hawaiian mythology,[14] there was originally one Source of all things. In order to create our current world and existence, the Source divided into three:

Kane – ruler of the above or upper world, aumakua, divine consciousness

Lono – ruler of the middle world, mental, conscious mind, considered the architect or builder of reality

Ku – ruler of the lower world, unconscious mind, physical incarnation

These rulers are also aligned with the worlds discussed earlier.

14 For additional information on the ancient Hawaiians, see: *An Account of The Polynesian Race: Its Origin and Migrations and Ancient History of the Hawaiian People to the Times of Kamehameha I* by Abraham Fornander, published by Charles E. Tuttle Company, ISBN 0804800022.

In the physical body, the ku is the lower-self that is concerned with physical body, memory and survival. It does not "think." It is like the hard drive of a computer in that it only holds ordinary and non-ordinary reality memories.[15] It cannot lie. The ku is also the gatekeeper to non-ordinary reality.

The middle-self is the lono. It is the mind that analyzes, guides the ku and gives instructions. As the analyzer, it sometimes gets in the way by over-analyzing situations and not trusting the information it is given from the ku. The middle-self provides a home for the ego.

The aumakua is the upper-self. As described above, the aumakua is the mother of intuition and influencer of the mental functions. Mental functions are fed information to the lono from the aumakua via the ku. The aumakua feeds the ku with "intuitive memories." Almost every person can recall an example of this communication. Do you remember a time that you "knew" information but could not recall how or why? This was the aumakua providing you with the data you needed at that time. The aumakua is the guide of our actions that has the benefit of knowing all things.

---

15 Dr. Wesselman uses computer-based terminology to bring the Shamanic theories into our modern speech in his book, *The Journey to the Sacred Garden: A Guide to Traveling in the Spiritual Realms*, published by Hay House, Inc., ISBN 1401901115. In this work, he describes how the percussive beat used by Shamans provides the "double-click" that allows access to the Shamanic realms.

Energies and Realities

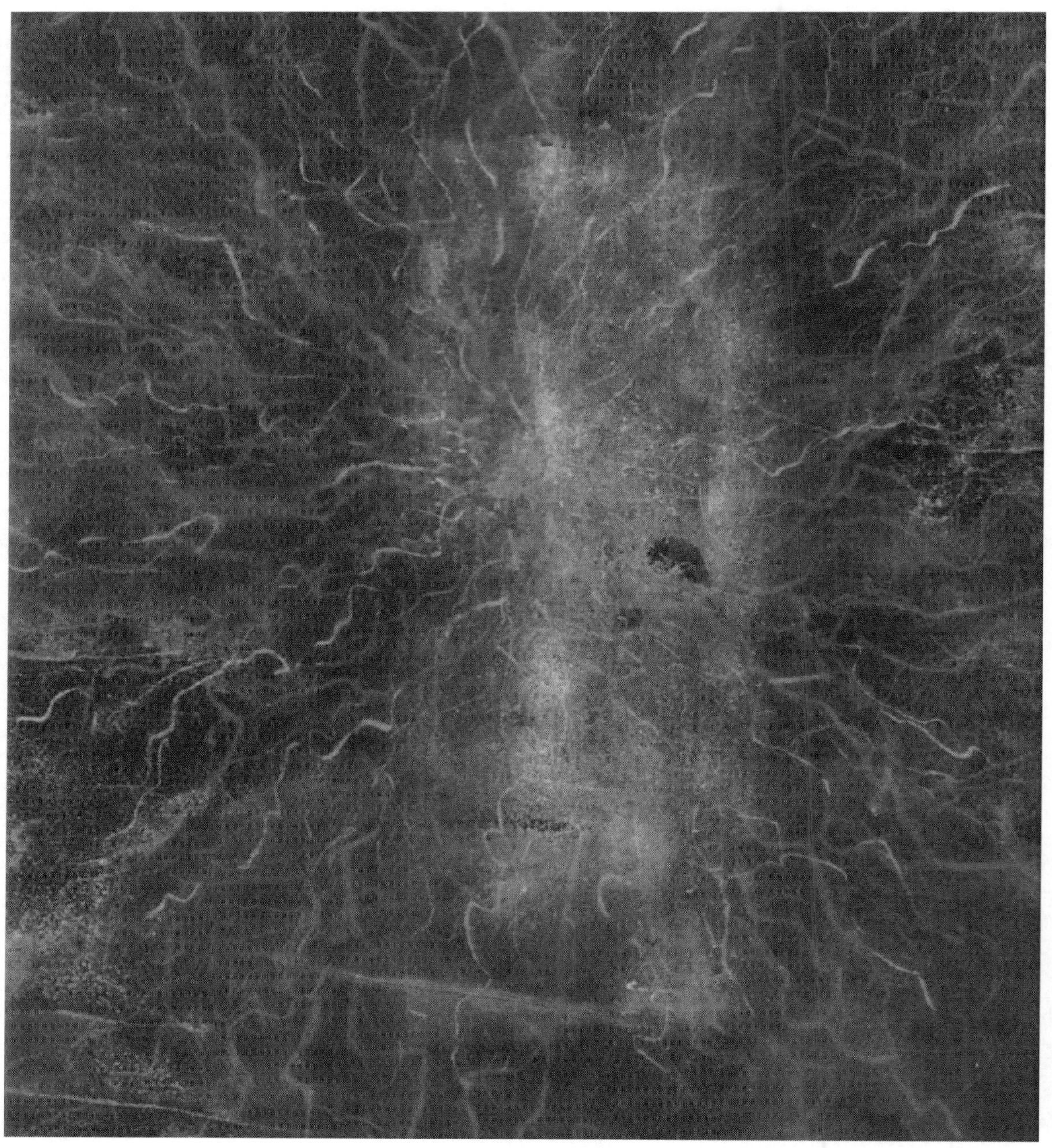

"Drawn to the Doorway" (negative image, detail)

Other realities and energy are around us all the time. We just need to learn how to see them.

In Shamanic practices, as we discussed earlier, there is the concept of ordinary and non-ordinary reality. The Shaman "rides" a beam of energy to non-ordinary reality to gather information that will be of benefit to his client.

I view the beam energy as the "carrier frequency"[16] that allows a person to connect to these worlds and realities. These energies, like the information in the Shaman's journey, are represented by symbols. Each symbol supports a specific aspect of reality or self and boosts the client's life force energy...enabling them to heal specific aspects of themselves.

There are physical and unconscious energies supporting the ku (or basic-self) that allow you to get in touch with the feeling of safety, unconscious fears, sexuality and knowledge that the body will be nourished.

Further, there are mental and conscious energies that empower the lono (or middle-self) to address compassion issues and acknowledge the aumakua (or higher-self.) Any issues of the mind or conscious change would be dealt with using this energy.

There is spiritual energy to support the aumakua or higher-self. This energy helps one to reconnect with the "Christ consciousness" (living life as a spiritual being in human form versus a human being having spiritual experiences.) It also helps one begin to understand the path of enlightenment. This energy can help you know your mission in this lifetime.

The synthesis of these energies, plus a balance of logic and intuition, allows direct connection with the Divine Source!

---

16 According to the online dictionary Wikipedia (http://en.wikipedia.org), carrier frequency is the frequency to which a receiver should be tuned in order to demodulate the information signal.

Dr. Hank Wesselman and many other Shamanic teachers describe two aspects of all the things in Shamanism: ordinary and non-ordinary. There appears to be a common tie between Shamanic teachings, Native American medicine wheel concepts and Kabbalistic practices that hints at the antiquity of these concepts. Kabbalistic practices describe concentric circles that allow the understanding of the souls. Rabbi David A. Cooper in *The Mystical Kabbalah*[17] describes the universes of the Kabbalah as concentric circles. I view the tie between the Shamanistic, Native American and Kabbalistic practices as follows:

Shamanic Reality/Aspect	Kabbalistic Soul Circles	Native American Medicine Wheel Symbology
Ordinary physical reality	Outer Ring – Existence, manifestation, time and space, physical world, ordinary reality	Earth – Dealing with the physical body, minerals, security
Non-ordinary physical reality (unconscious)	Middle-Outer Ring – Creation, speech, emotions, "different" reality	Water – Covering the emotions, trust, innocence, fear
Ordinary conscious mind	Middle-Inner Ring – Intellect, formation of thoughts, places where time does not exist, higher realms, angelic planes	Fire – Human spirit, pleasure, beauty
Non-ordinary conscious mind	–	–
Ordinary spiritual	Inner Ring – Emanation, archetypes, life force, living essence of creation	Air – Wisdom, knowledge, elder, stars
Non-ordinary spiritual	Center Point – Primordial Being from which all life sprung, unity, connection with the Divine	Center Point – Whole, balanced, Great Spirit, unity

17 *The Mystical Kabbalah* (Audio Edition) by Rabbi David A. Cooper, published by Sounds True, ISBN 1564557294

Similar correlations can be made with the energies and/or symbolism used in Ancient Rainbow Conscious Healing. These are described on Laurie Grant's web site and in her seminars. (See http://www.archhealing.com.)

One aspect not specifically addressed by Native Americans or Kabbalists is the concept of the non-ordinary conscious mind. I see this as the trance state that Shamans and healing practitioners achieve where they are able to transcend ordinary reality and comprehend the spirit world.

As you can see, the description of the souls as practiced by Kabbalists is very similar to the practices of Shamans and Native Americans. We will discuss these commonalities in a later chapter.

I would like to relate a story that dramatically illustrates our innate ability to utilize the specific frequencies of energy that support our physical body...we just forget how. Recently, my son and I were relaxing and my mind drifted to a problem with which I had been wrestling. For some reason, my son turned quickly with a worried look in his eyes and said, "What's wrong?" Although I had given no physical clues, my son picked up on my anxiety.

From my work as an energy healer, I have become attuned to the different frequencies that my clients are absorbing. These energies can be broadly classified as physical or mental/emotional. When my son experienced the emotion of concern for my well-being, I felt an immediate and powerful rush of mental/emotional energy course through his body. Although I was touching him at the time, I was not consciously attempting to facilitate any type of energy transference or healing work. My son, quite naturally, had drawn the proper frequency that his body needed to cope with his fear or concern for me.

Children <u>know</u> that they are one with the Divine. They are constantly accessing this Divine Energy flow. They use this energy, mostly unconsciously, to support and nurture their bodies. This support allows them to stay grounded and to deal with situations as they manifest.

This instinctive knowledge is present in all of us. We just forget how to use it or we have the knowledge suppressed by parents, elders, teachers or societal norms that do not reinforce our intuition. When we forget how to access and use the Divine Source Energy to feed our physical and emotional bodies, our energy stores are depleted – leading to illness, depression, anxiety and many of the ailments found in today's highly stressful lifestyles.

Chapter 3: Religions

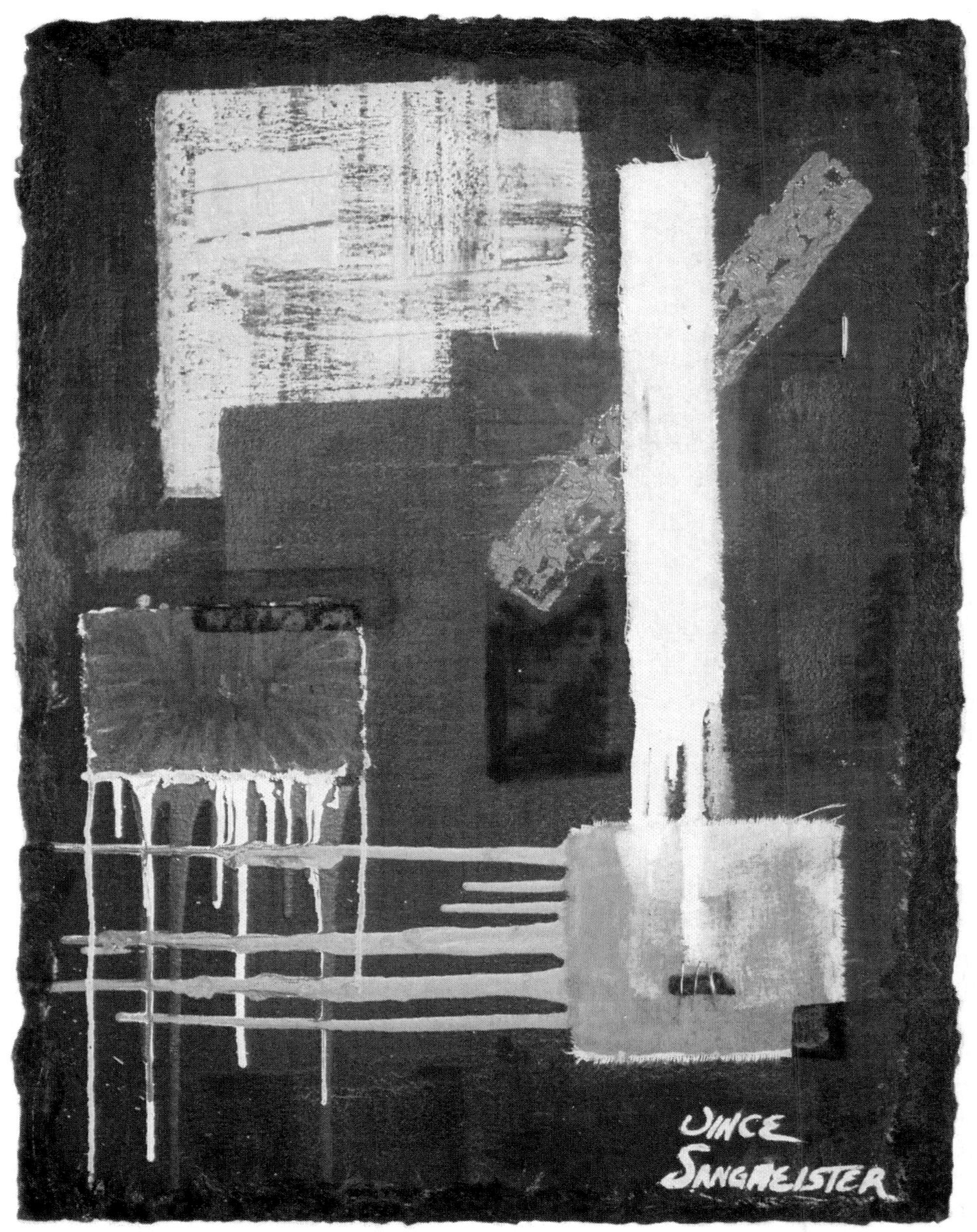

"Heaven, Earth and Between"

We spend lifetimes trying to fill the void between Heaven and Earth.

Heaven is a palace with many doors
And each may enter in his own way...
- Hindu saying

One of my clients was raised Lutheran her whole life and clearly remembers sitting through sermons each Sunday. However, she does not remember the subject of any of the sermons. She did not believe that she had heard one word of the message in over 50 years of going to church. After her energy-healing treatments, however, she said that for the first time, she had gone to church and heard the message.

The religious practices you have participated in probably have brought you great comfort and joy. They have provided security for you – and served you well, perhaps. If they have succeeded in reconnecting you, truly, with the Divine Source, then honor these practices...be thankful for them.

However, if they have obscured your view to the path of Oneness, then once again, I suggest that you re-examine how your practices, religious or otherwise, can be aligned with the Oneness principles discussed earlier.

In this chapter, you will see how:

- Practices of ancient civilizations promoted a direct connection with the Divine Source
- Changing the focus of your prayers can make a huge impact on everything from your daily life to worldwide issues

Questions answered for me in this chapter include:

- Is Oneness a new concept?
- Why now?
- How can we use the gift of Oneness energy?

Direct Connection

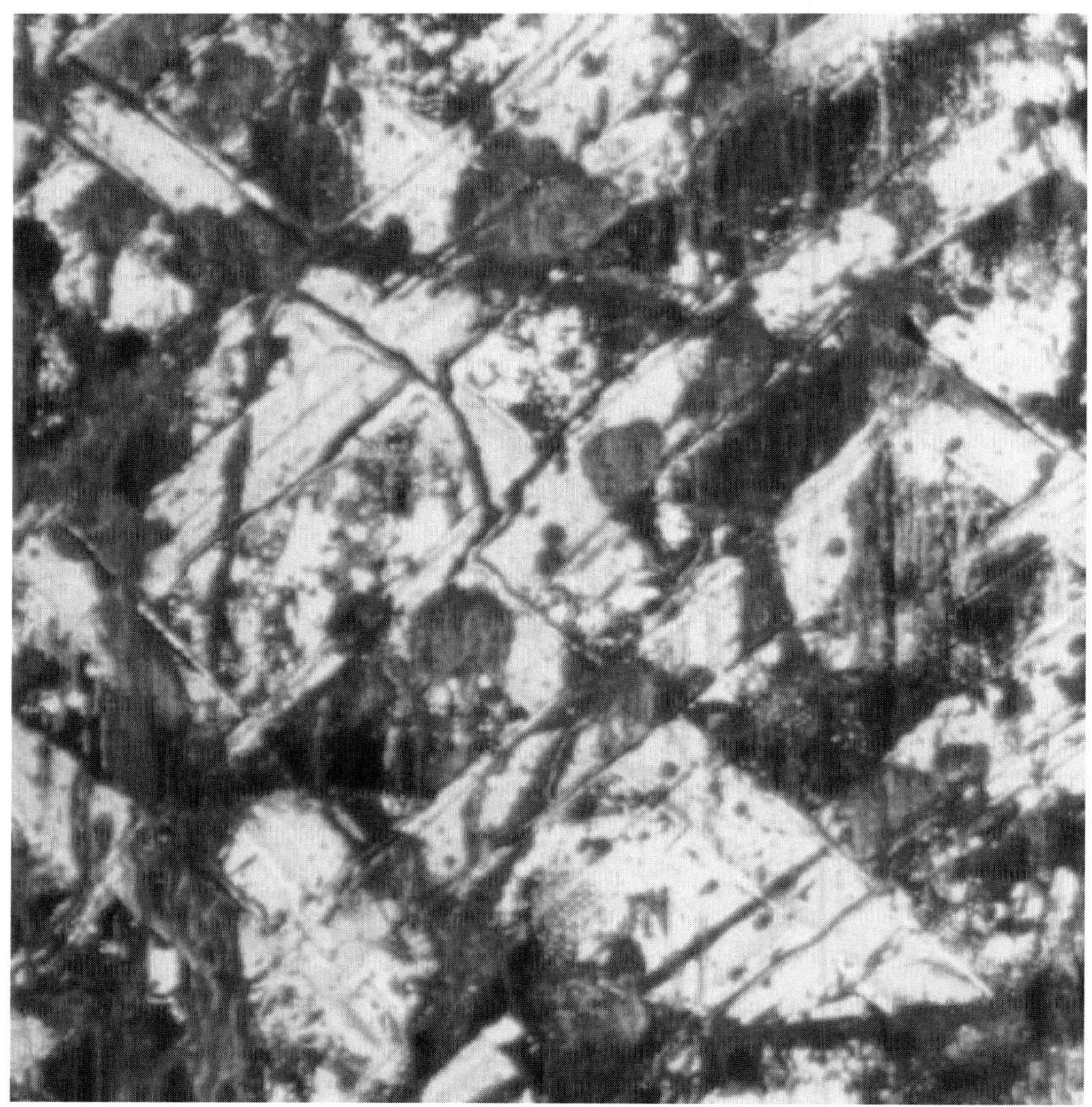

"Blue Agony Resurrection" (detail)

A web ties the forms of energy together...Connecting us all to each other and the Divine.

The early Hawaiian religious beliefs were much the some as early Christianity. No hierarchy (bishop, archbishop, cardinal, pope, minister, deacon, etc.) was needed between the worshiper and the Source. We see this concept in Christianity in the book of Mark, chapter 10:42-45:

> 42But Jesus called them to Himself and said to them, "You know that those who are considered rulers over the Gentiles lord it over them, and their great ones exercise authority over them. 43Yet it shall not be so among you, but whoever desires to become great among you shall be your servant. 44And whoever of you desires to be first shall be slave of all. 45For even the Son of Man did not come to be served, but to serve, and to give His life as a ransom for many."

This passage shows that the original Christian beliefs did not want the "leaders" to be placed on a pedestal above the common man. True leaders are the servant of man helping their brothers and sisters reconnect with the Divine. This connection is available to all of us.

The ancient Hawaiians, as best as can be determined, were not unlike the first Americans. They honored the earth and its bounties. They showed their thanks through prayer, offerings and a reverence for all things. They saw the divine hand in all. They were one with the land and their God!

Earlier, we talked about the Hawaiian belief that all things are part of the Divine Source. This is in sharp contrast to the normal actions and beliefs associated with many of the world's religions. Many of these belief systems insist that they are the only path to the Divine and that if you are not a member of their sect, you are going to "Hell." This dualistic "us and them" approach has been a factor in nearly every war that has ever been fought since the days of Cain and Abel.

I find it bizarre that some people are willing to kill you because you do not believe in their concept of what happens after you die.

It is time to heal the split between man and the Divine that occurred so many years ago and that causes so much suffering today.

There could not be a better time than right now. Many researchers and prophets consider this time in history as a great awakening – a time when humans begin to understand their full capacities. Many of the seers look to the 26,000-year cycle of our solar system as it transits the Milky Way Galaxy and see signs that this time in history is an era of enlightenment.

The ancient Mayan calendar, which tracks this 26,000-year cycle with astonishing accuracy, ends in 2012 AD and predicts the end of the world, as we know it. Some people would look at these times with fear; foreseeing catastrophic earth changes and social upheaval. Others who can see and live in the light believe that we have a wonderful opportunity to:

– participate in a large scale reawakening to new levels of consciousness,

– make a quantum leap on our path of enlightenment, and

– reconnect with the Divine Source!

Modern Mayan Shamans are also speaking and writing on the importance of this time. Carlos Barrios, Mayan historian, anthropologist and investigator, speaks of this time in which we are living as a time of transformation.[18] The year 2012 is not an ending, but a beginning. This will be a time of transformation from a materialistic world to an era where peace is the norm and people live in harmony with each other and Mother Earth.

In his book, *The Flower of Life,*[19] Drunvalo Melchizedek talks about the Great Year, which is the 26,000-year cycle of our solar system. He suggests that the keepers of ancient knowledge encoded the keys necessary to understand the secrets of the universe. He believes that this time in our history is a great awakening after a 13,000-year sleep.

This implies that we "went to sleep" approximately 13,000-years ago. Graham Hancock in his video series *Quest for the Lost Civilization,*[20] offers evidence that great monuments around the globe, including Egypt's Great Pyramid, Cambodia's Angkor Wat and Mexico's Tiahuanaco were constructed 12,500 years ago, contrary to commonly accepted theories. I find the similarities in time very interesting. These monuments could hold the "encoded keys" that our ancestors left for us to discover when it was time.

As with any change, this time will not be smooth sailing. It is human nature to resist change. Many of you may remember a cigarette commercial from the 1970's that said, "I'd rather fight than switch." Many people who cannot grow and evolve into this new world will fight, die and potentially take others with them. An example of this type of resistance would be when a leader's goal is that "his organization" is still in existence 100 years from now without regard for the souls who make up the organization. Such a leader would not care if those people are gone, sacrificed or disillusioned to the point of complacency.

---

18 See *Kam Wuj El Libro del Destino*, by Carlos Barios and Ludovica Squirru, published by Sudamericana, ISBN 9500714493.

19 *The Ancient Secret of the Flower of Life: Volumes 1 and 2* by Drunvalo Melchizedek, published by Light Technology Publications, ISBN 1891824171 and 189182421X.

20 *Quest for the Lost Civilization* (video) starring Graham Hancock, published by Acorn Media, ASIN 1569382603.

As you look at the world's belief systems and strip away the culture, dogma and politics, several basic universal truths that support the theory of a common understanding become evident:

There is one true Source that created all!

Love your neighbor and all that you encounter!

Respect nature!

Be thankful!

These truths have a central theme that can be summed up as **Love** and **Compassion**. In this model, your "enemy" is a reflection of you. Your desire to kill that enemy is your desire to remove that part of you that you <u>will</u> <u>not</u> or <u>cannot</u> acknowledge. This concept is true for both negative and positive traits. You cannot love your enemy unless you love yourself.

Remember one of the Oneness/Aikido principles: If you attempt to "see the world from your enemy's eyes," you begin to have compassion for his or her situation and experience the world without bias.

In Aikido, the true art is moving within your own space regardless of what your uke (partner) is doing. It teaches you to be true to your own path while acknowledging there are other paths. In an effort to halt your progress, the uke will grab, or over extend and cause an awakening. The uke is offered the ability to see the world through your eyes or to experience the consequences. Either way, you are true to your path.

Your happiness is not what others think, observe, or do. Happiness is **your** manifestation of **your** life in a way that is beneficial to **you**. Live your life based on your actions – not the actions of another that displease, offend or cause you grief. Accept that the person is fulfilling his or her path outlined by the Source. In the words of William Shakespeare, "All the world is a stage and all the men and women are merely players."[21] This goes a long way toward understanding that, in life, like in the body, someone has to be the heart cell and someone has to be the cancer cell. We all, at one time or another, had to be the cancer cell so that the heart cell may grow and flourish.

As you remove cultural influences from the world's religious teachings, the story is the same: There is but one GOD, Source, Yahweh, Great Spirit, IAO – The invisible force that holds everything together. Reconnect with that Source directly and you are on your true path – what an awesome life you will live!

Some people have a problem with "invisible forces" guiding their lives. However, we live with invisible forces all the time: gravity, electricity and UV light. All are invisible but

21 From *As You Like It* by William Shakespeare.

are real and demonstrate their presence regularly. Recent findings from the National Aeronautics and Space Administration (NASA) Wilkinson Microwave Anisotropy Probe (WMAP) indicate that over 70% of the known universe is made of "Dark Energy."[22] According to the NASA results, the energy appears as a "universal constant."

The Source is no different. There is a beautiful saying: "A rose by any other name would smell as sweet."[23] If you call the wind "Dave," would it blow any differently? Nearly all religions carry the belief in One Supreme Being; the name is only our way of quantifying the un-quantifiable.

Is it possible that the "universal constant" found by WMAP is the co-creative energy provided by the Source?

Science has many methods for identifying, classifying, documenting and explaining energy. When the explanation is not quick in coming or is beyond our ability to comprehend, it is called faith or imagined. The bottom line is that the energy that makes up humans, the cosmos and all that we can ever hope to discover is part of the Divine Source Energy.

---

22 See http://map.gsfc.nasa.gov for further information on the WMAP mission.
23 From *Romeo and Juliet* by William Shakespeare.

Prayer

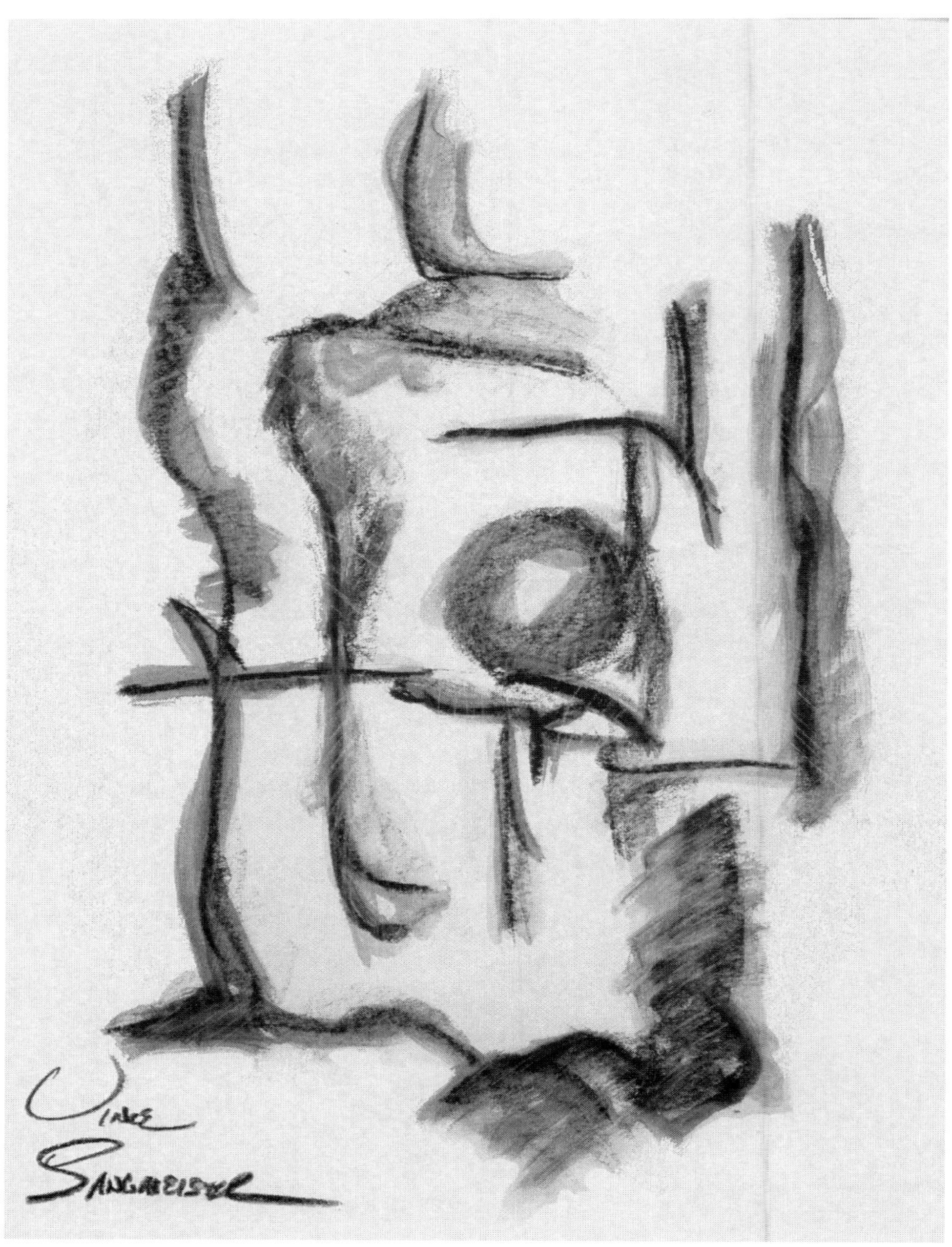

"Solitary Man"

Prayer: The solitary, personal act of direct connection to the Divine.

Another key aspect of spirituality, religions and Oneness, is prayer. When we pray, we attempt to quantify the invisible chain between man and the Source. For the most part, we do not make prayer part of our daily lives. We are "overtaken by events" and "just too busy."

Too busy to honor and connect with what we so strongly want / need to understand?

When we do pray, we tend to pray with negative emotions as our focus. On his tape, "*The Lost Mode of Prayer*,"[24] Gregg Braden describes that a prayer is a thought, feeling and emotion that we charge with Divine Source Energy in order to manifest our wishes or desires. Normally, we have prayers like:

> "I pray that it rains..."
>
> "Please God, don't let this happen..."
>
> "I pray for a better job..."

In each of these examples, the underlying emotion is fear. Fear that there will not be enough rain for the crops, fear that something that we consider "bad" is going to happen, fear that our job is inadequate. The emotion of fear is in direct conflict with some of the "basic universal truths" described earlier.

Instead, we should be "positively" co-creating with the Divine Source in our prayers. We should take the energy that the Source is constantly providing, use this energy to fill our prayer with "mana" (or "life force") and send our wish to the world around us. Remember how our thoughts, feelings and emotions impact the world around us? Since our prayers are a very powerful medium for transmitting this information, we need to ensure that we send them with positive energy.

So, how do we do this?

We change the emotion associated with the prayer. For example, healers and Shamans in ancient Egypt and Greece, in modern day China and in Ancient Rainbow Conscious Healing, will focus on seeing the ailment as already healed. This is the kind of focus that we need to place in our prayers.

In doing so, our prayers take on a form that is different than we are used to. This type of prayer concentrates positive energy into our thought form. Using this method, our "rain" prayer becomes:

> In my mind, I sense how the ground smells after the rain, how the cool grass feels under my feet, and I see all the things I can do with the perfect amount of water.

---

24 Listen to *The Lost Mode of Prayer* by Gregg Braden, published by Sounds True, ISBN 1564556670.

Next, you would increase the "mana" in these thoughts with the energy from the Source. You then express your gratitude to the Source for the abundance...and send the prayer off to manifest.

This model can be used for any prayer. This is true co-creation.

Besides keeping our thoughts, feelings and emotions positive when praying, there is another very important thought to keep in mind. In prayer, one is attempting to contact the Divine, but we tend to do all the talking. The Spirit of all spirits is the creator of the all that we can see, envision, dream of, speculate on or imagine. The Divine is the creator of all that we cannot see or ever hope to develop the mental capacity to understand. Does it not seem pretentious for us to do all the talking during the prayer? Remember to listen to the Divine when praying. It may just be a bee buzzing around your head, but the bee is one of the Divine's creations also. The Divine speaks to us through all creation.

Co-creation goes back a long way.

Each and every one of us agreed to the goal of our life's work in this existence. As taught in Laurie Grant's seminars and in Dr. Wesselman's book *Journey to the Sacred Garden: A Guide to Traveling in the Spiritual Realms*,[25] we all met with our personal cosmic council of elders prior to incarnating to discuss this lifetime. Like a good business plan, we outlined what we would accomplish, what our requirements were, what help and skills we would need, etc. The Council helped us to develop this plan and an agreement or contract was signed by all present. The Council also watches over our progress and helps us.

My contract is responsible for this book.

Have you ever had a nagging feeling that you are not doing what you are supposed to be doing? Your job is not satisfying? Regrets over a decision?

25 Laurie teaches about the council of elders in her classes. A similar "council" theory is also addressed in Dr. Wesselman's book, *The Journey to the Sacred Garden: A Guide to Traveling in the Spiritual Realms*, published by Hay House, Inc., ISBN 1401901115.

Take note of these feelings and thoughts. It may not necessarily mean that you should quit your job and sail around the world. Maybe those inklings have something to teach you. Perhaps they are offering information that you need to accomplish your goal and fulfill your contract?

Listen to your heart! Feel the connection with the Divine plan. Ask for help!

Recognize that we are never alone when we truly co-create.

Co-create in Oneness!

Everyday Miracles

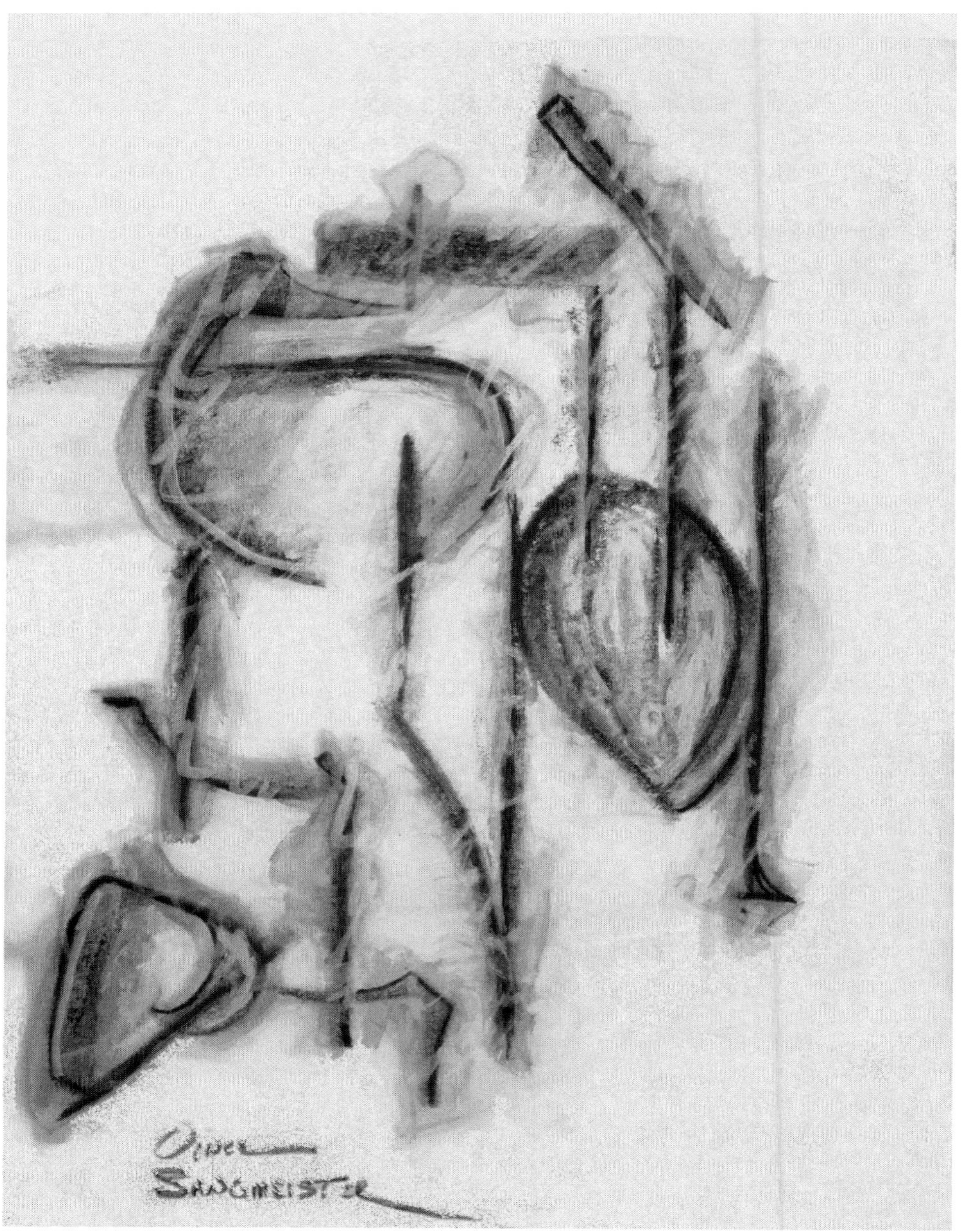

"Coeur"

Coeur or heart...the beating of the miracle of life that we can connect with any time.

Oneness and connection with the Divine Source are not just tools for one-on-one interaction. It allows us to tap into the carrier frequency of the Divine Source Energy.

Co-create!

These energies can be directed to just about any situation...your job, family, environment, health, etc. Always remember to:

> Bring your spirit helpers and guides with you. You will find that everyone you encounter is a "friend."
>
> Ask for guidance. You are never alone.
>
> Seek the knowledge that will allow all parties involved to feel like they were represented and equitable decisions were made.
>
> See, truly understand and be thankful for the "other" point of view.
>
> Know that the people with whom you interact are striving to fulfill their contract as well. Treat their paths with respect. Purposefully standing in their way is not fostering the spiritual growth of you or them.
>
> Be thankful for rain, even when it is the driest.
>
> Be thankful for the sun, when it rains.
>
> Be thankful!

As an example, many of us have seen people in the street asking for money or food. Regardless of your opinion of the person's authenticity, the common reaction is to ignore the person and rationalize that you do not have any spare change or that you are in a hurry.

Consider this as an alternative...

Pray that they understand their Divine path and feel their Oneness.

This simple act may not put food in their mouths, but, as we have seen before, the positive thought, feeling and emotion that you charge with Divine Source Energy can fill this person as no food can.

Chapter 4: Oneness Healing

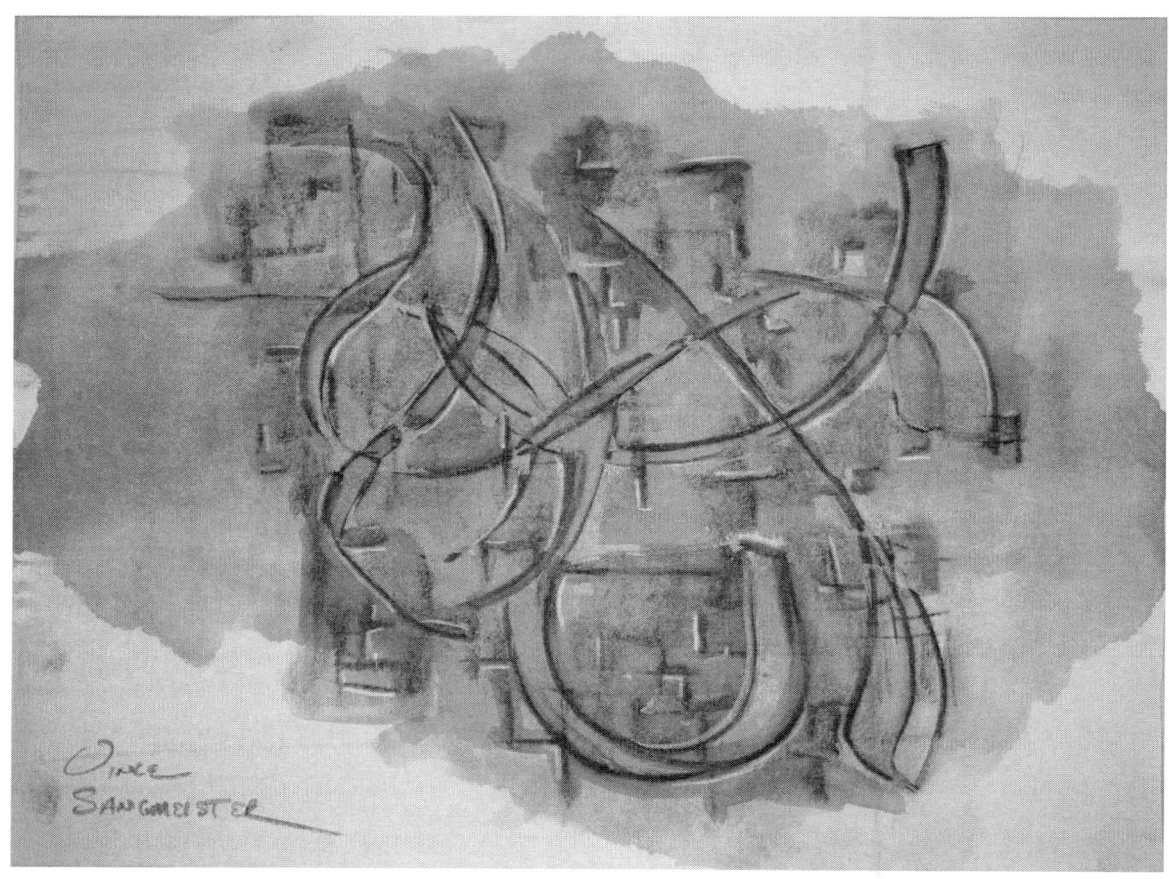

"Metropolitan Vortices"

Our "real" world...full of the lines of energy that we offer to our environment with the ever-present rainbow of energy from the Divine.

First we receive the light, then we impart it. Thus we repair the world.
- Kabbalah

I was working in my basement office when the babysitter said that there was a bird in the fireplace. I went up to look and saw the bird flapping behind the glass doors. I got my motorcycle gauntlets for protection and went to get the bird out. When I looked closely, I was amazed to see that the bird was a young, red-tailed hawk. I was shocked that such an intelligent bird had gotten stuck in such an embarrassing situation! I centered myself and connected with the hawk's spirit. I explained that I was not going to hurt him, just help him to return to freedom. To my pleasure and amazement, the hawk turned its back to me and calmed down. I opened the glass doors and screens, placed a towel over the hawk, picked it up and took it outside. I placed the hawk on the ground and uncovered it. It remained on the ground for a few minutes while it caught its breath. It then flew off and perched in a tree, shaken, but uninjured.

This amazing experience showed me how far the concepts of Oneness and connectivity to the Source really reach. They encompass all life forces in this realm (humans, animals, etc.) and beyond (spirits, angels, guides, etc.) Then I started realizing that just knowing about these concepts and believing in them is not enough. I needed to practice them – everyday, every moment, every situation.

In doing this, we will all heal...we will make miracles happen everyday...we will help others and ourselves. This is true Oneness healing.

In this chapter, you will be introduced to:

- the aka web and its role in connecting us all
- how a healer can help achieve Oneness through this web connection
- the chakra system and its role in healing

A question answered for me in this chapter: How does a healer use the Oneness connection to assist the healing process?

We are All Connected

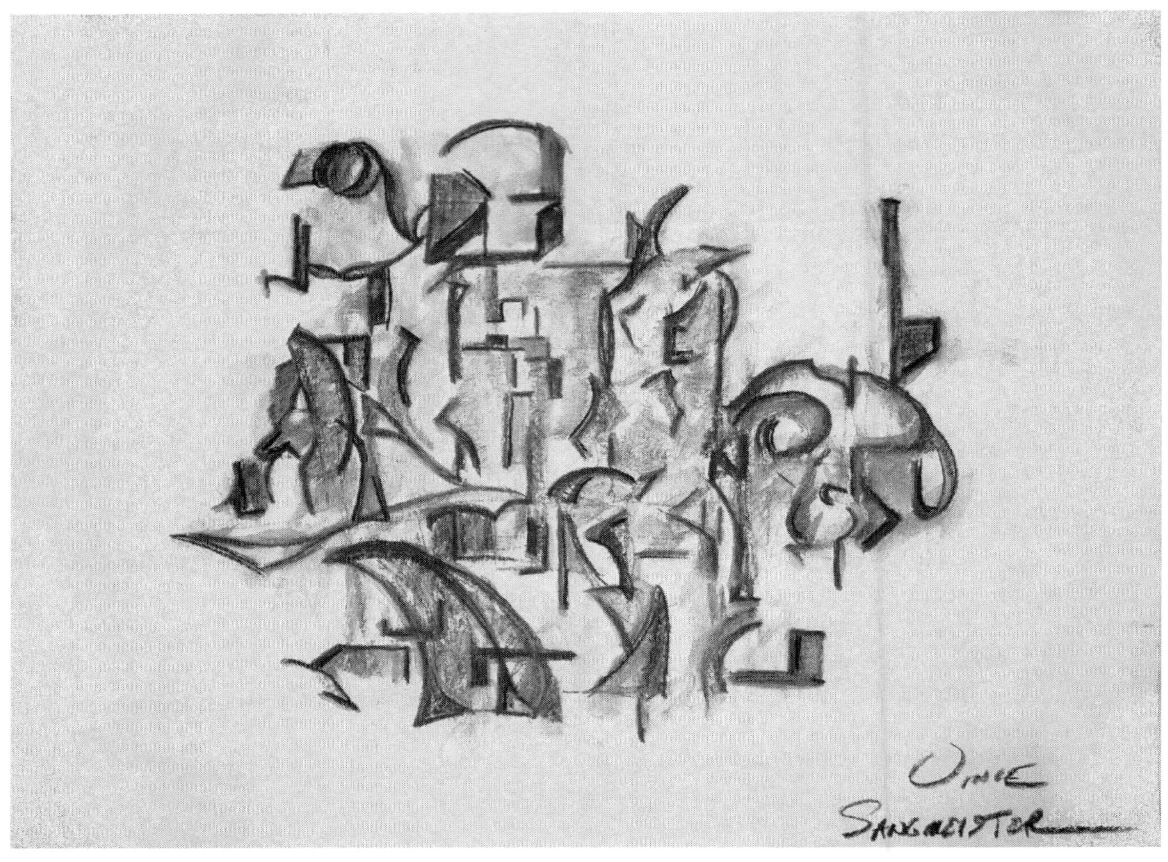

"Fractured Self"

Although the thread of connection may be thin…it is possible to see everything as One…made up of connections…sometimes thinner than a spider's web, but still, connected.

In the teachings of Gregg Braden,[26] Hank Wesselman,[27] Laurie Grant[28] and indigenous peoples, we find a shared common connection that the Hawaiians call the aka web. During my mediations, I have traveled this web, connecting with other "nodes" to heal, be healed and gain knowledge. In order to understand the aka web, one must go back to the beginning of existence, to the "Big Bang." This instant in time was not a colossal explosion of matter. It was an expanding of consciousness.

This consciousness formed what we see and experience now. All that we see, all the matter in the universe as we know it, is what this consciousness understood – it needed to grow and develop. Everything in the universe is part of this consciousness. Many times, we look at a plant, for example, and think that it is not "conscious" by our definition. It is not that the plant is not conscious; it is only that we do not have a point of reference to comprehend the consciousness of the plant.

There are many consciousnesses that we do not understand at this point in our development. We cannot communicate with these consciousnesses because we do not have an understanding of the thoughts, feelings and emotions that the "foreign" consciousness has.

It is similar to being in a dark room where you can hear someone speaking in a foreign language. The words are alien. The context is unknown. You are pretty sure that the person is trying to communicate with you or someone else. Your mind, however, does not have a base-level knowledge of how to communicate or if you are even part of the communication. Therefore, the message is lost.

When a healer connects to the aka web, it is possible to communicate with all entities without necessarily having an understanding of the underlying "language" of thoughts, feelings and emotions. Also, through the web, one is able to receive help from entities that might be considered alien or foreign to his or her comprehension.

The aka web is not a linear spider's web. It is a three-dimensional lattice that resembles the patterns observed in a crystalline solid. The web allows us to break through the walls of misunderstanding that we might have built by allowing a direct spiritual connection to the Divine and to each other.

---

26 Gregg Braden discussed this connection in his presentation at The Prophet's Conference in Santa Fe, New Mexico, June 2002.

27 In Dr. Wesselman's book, *Visionseeker: Shared Wisdom from the Place of Refuge* (published by Hay House, Inc., ISBN 1561707538), he describes a Shamanic journey to this web.

28 As taught in Laurie's seminars. See http://www.archhealing.com.

When a Shaman or healer works with a client, the Shaman is helping the client to receive and direct the Source energy. The Shaman understands and works under the basic knowledge that we are all connected via the aka web. The thoughts, feelings and emotions of each and every one of us form "nodes" on the web that allow us to share a common bond. The aka web permits an exchange of information and energies at a higher vibrational level than would be possible on the physical plane.

Achieving Oneness with a Healer

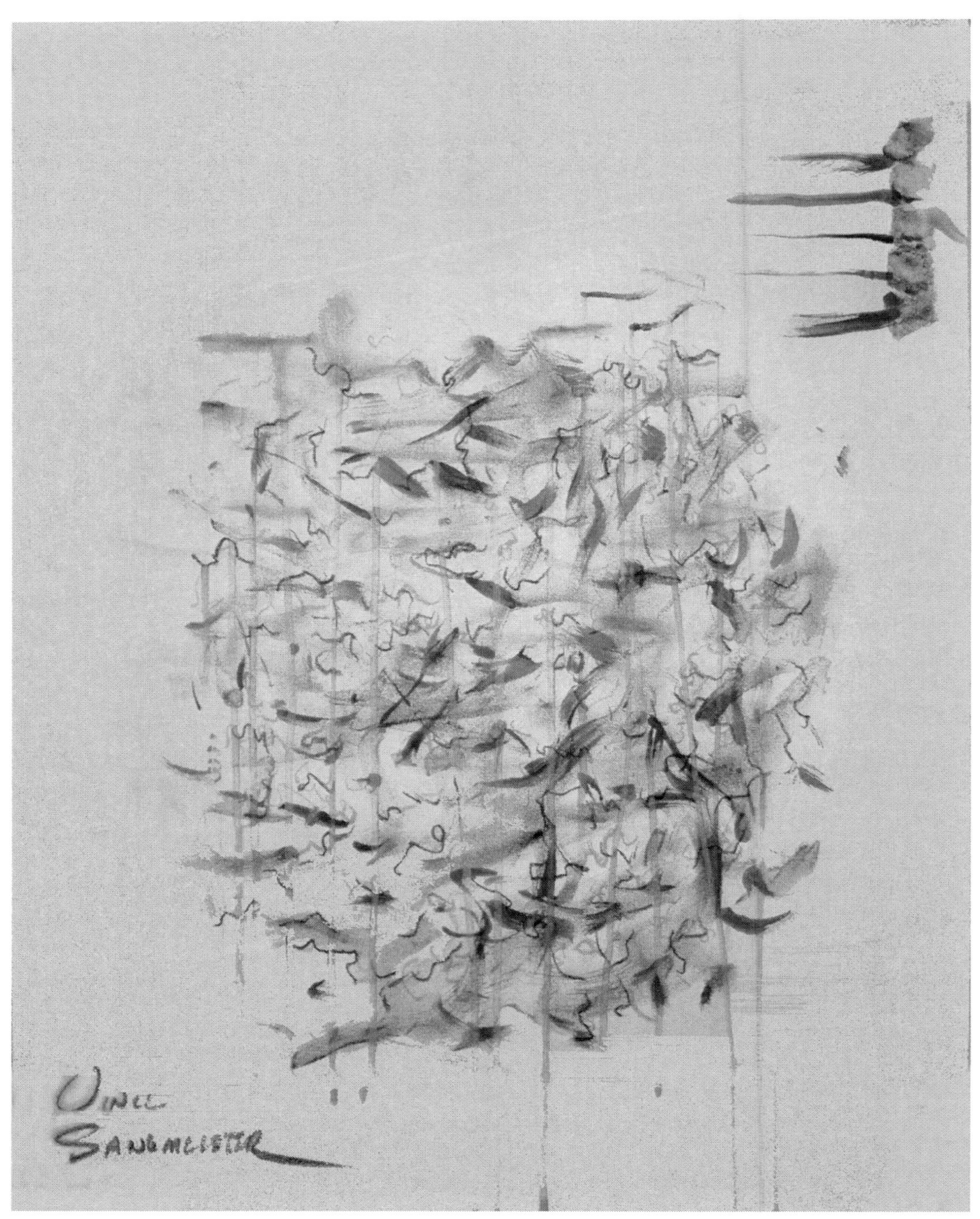

"Active"

Searching for the connection, our paths cross many that can help us on our journey.

As a healing session begins, Shamans will connect with their node of the aka web in order to expand their consciousness. This facilitates the connection with the client's node. The healing energies will then be directed to the client via the web connections. The web provides the conduit or medium over which the energy is carried. By using the web as the conduit, Shamans can augment their focus with the positive energies of all entities that wish to help guide healing energy to the client. Additionally, any of the client's own spiritual energy that might be available on other vibrational levels can be used.

This technique allows the Shaman to open more energy channels than might be readily available if the healing were attempted strictly on the physical plane. Even though the physical connection might be powerful, the aka web connection joins not only the Shaman and client, but also binds all entities to each other and to the Divine Source. The aka connection will therefore be far stronger and will transcend time – giving the client the ability to heal in the past, present and potentially future.

A Shaman will strive to use a level of energy that is beneficial to the client and the Shaman. By using the web, which is at a higher vibration to begin with, the client can absorb the highest vibration that is beneficial to his or her spirit, mind and body. It is also very important that the Shaman only facilitate a level of energy that is to his/her benefit in addition to the client. (There are many Shamans and healers in the world today, sometimes referred to as "wounded healers," that cause harm to themselves by trying to facilitate an energy connection that is beyond their capability to process.)

The Divine Source Energy, tapped from the web via a Shaman or healer, helps clients build their reserves of mana. The term "mana" has the meaning "water" in Hawaii and other Polynesian cultures – but it also means the "life force energy" that ties all things to the Divine Source. The mana acts like the water that allows one to germinate and grow the seed of one's dream. Without water, a seed is dormant, yet alive and ready to develop. When water is added, the seed germinates and grows into a completely different organism at a higher energy level. Additionally, this one seed holds the information necessary to create more seeds in an ongoing process of growth and renewal.

Divine Source Energy is the water that allows all of us to grow from seeds to our higher vibrational potential. Shamanic and/or healing practices can facilitate the germination of seeds – be they optimal health, complete healing or peace on earth.

Healing Treatments

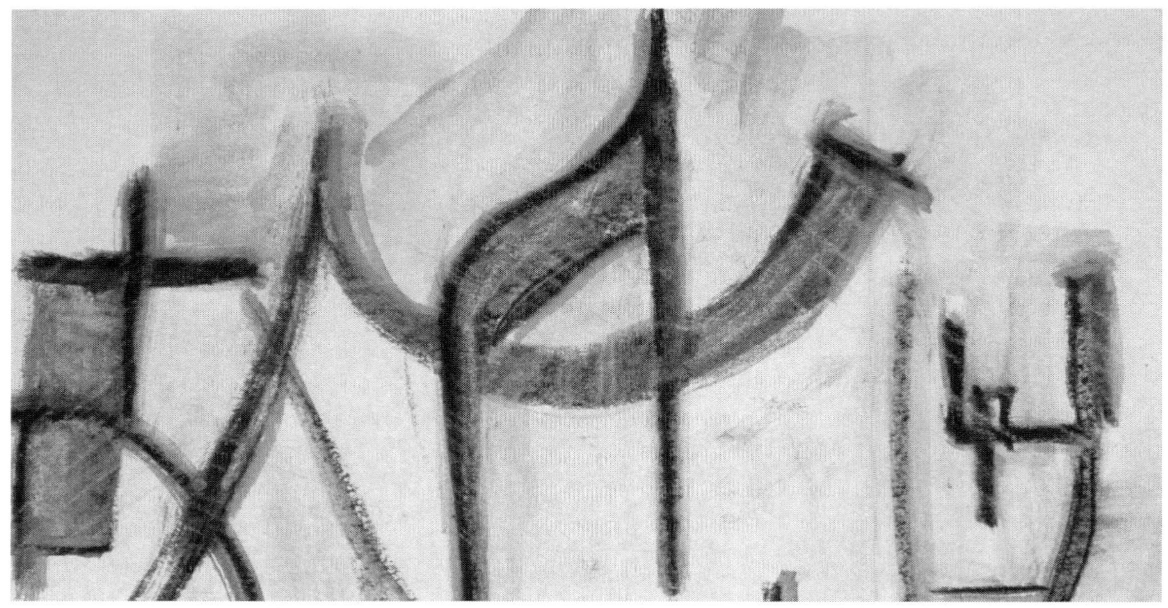

***"The Attempt (To Heal)"* (detail)**

Building the healing bridge...reconnecting with creation...this is the job of the healer.

I would now like to provide an example of how a healer addresses an ailment that is affecting his client using the concepts of Oneness. There are many other options that enable the client to experience and work with Divine Source Energy. You, as the healer or one being healed, should find the modality/path that most resonates with you and allows you to experience the full benefits of Oneness.

For me, energy healing is a spiritual path for both the client and myself. The energy provides a conduit that reconnects with the Divine and enables both the healer and client to see the world as Divine. I find that the energy healing practices of the Shaman resonate most with me.

To facilitate the healing, the Shaman will discuss the situation with the person and ask spirit guides for assistance. This discussion could be as simple as asking the person to state the aliment to be worked on, to as complex as a full history of the situation. The objective of the discussion is to identify any patterns that might help the healer or the client to pinpoint the root cause of the disharmony. These questions would progress along the line of:

> What would you like to heal?
>
> When did it first appear?
>
> What was happening in your life when it first appeared?
>
> Are there times when the disharmony appears more often or stronger?
>
> Has anyone in your family had a similar ailment?
>
> Are you aware of any lesson associated with the ailment?

At then end of the discussion, the healer will ask if the client is willing to accept the lesson. Acceptance of the situation, even if the lesson is not known to the client, is the key to beginning the healing process. Acceptance does not mean giving up. Acceptance, in this context, is acknowledgement. If a person is not willing to learn the lesson, the ailment is still "of use" to the client. Actually knowing the lesson is not necessarily essential for the healing to take place. The heart-felt acknowledgement of the situation is the most important aspect.

The client will then be directed to see the healing as already done. The process of seeing the healing in this way can be likened to the Shamanic practice of shape shifting. Traditionally, shape shifting is when a Shaman blends with or "becomes" something outside his or her normal physical form. This could be a plant, animal, tree, rock, etc. The shape will be chosen based on the information to be gathered. In healing, the client is directed to "shape shift" from an entity that is sick into a healthy form.

To accomplish this, the client will need to visualize all of the thoughts, feelings and emotions that are part of the ailment: how it feels (pain, cold, heat, numb, etc.), how it looks (disfigured, inflamed, scaly, red, etc.), how it sounds (ringing in the ears, moaning, screams, etc.), how it smells (infectious, acrid, pungent, etc.) and how it tastes (sickeningly sweet, dry, wet, stale, etc.). After thanking the ailment for the lesson it provided, the client would be asked to visualize a violet or white flame. This flame is not destructive like normal fire. It is loving and kind and contains intelligence far beyond our comprehension. The aspects of the ailment would be allowed to drift toward the flame. As it approaches the flame, it will be absorbed back into the collective energy system that nourishes all things.

After this is done, the client should then "shape shift" to a healthy entity by visualizing all of the thoughts, feelings and emotions that make up this healthy entity. This information will be the focused intention of the client throughout the healing session. During the session, the client will be instructed to keep his or her mind open to any thoughts, feelings, or emotions that manifest, acknowledge them, take note and allow them to pass.

After gathering the information and focusing the client's intention, the Shaman sets his or her intention on the information. Then, the Shaman enters the non-ordinary state of reality and travels to the appropriate worldly level to gather the information necessary to deal with the situation. To enter the non-ordinary state, the Shaman will normally use a percussive beat. The source of this beat could be a drum, rattle, didgeridoo, singing bowl, chanting, etc. The Shaman may "extract" imbalances from the client or bring something back from non-ordinary reality that is useful to the client like a power animal or soul part.

After returning from the journey, the Shaman will pass the information about the journey to the client.

Chakras

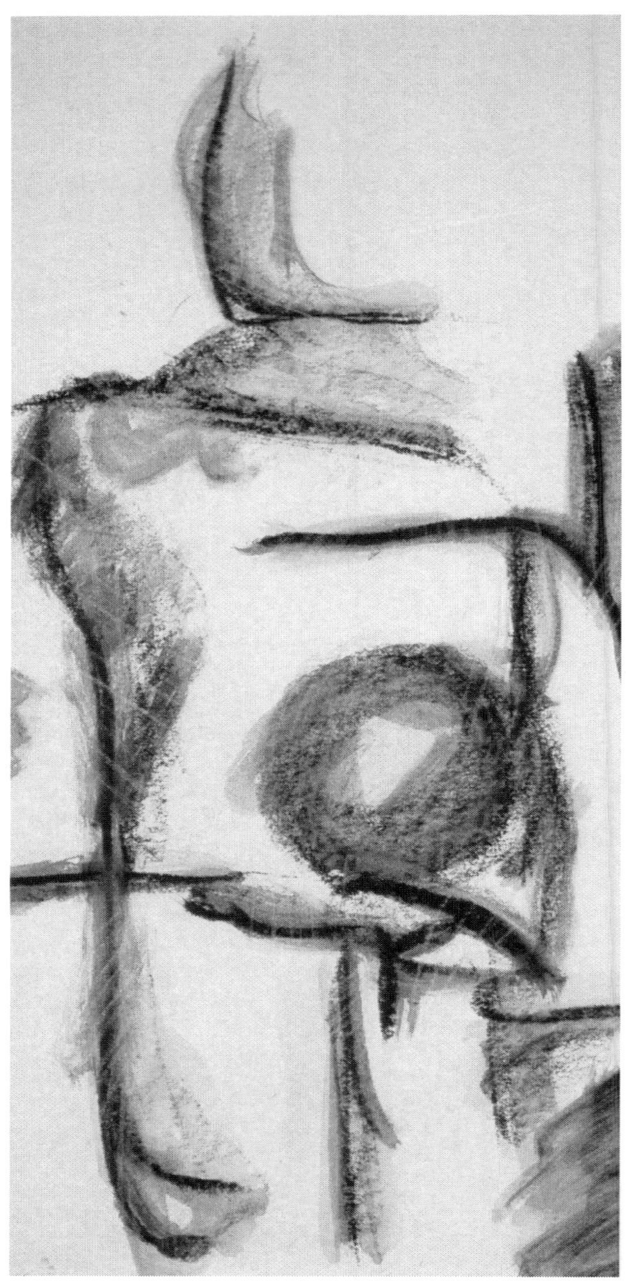

"Solitary Man" (detail)

The bodies that we are living inside of are miracles that need nurturing...the Chakras provide a place to store our energy reserves.

You have been hearing a lot about the role of energy in Oneness healing, so now it is time to discuss the role of charkas in the integration of this energy.

For the benefit of the readers who might not be familiar with the primary or bodily chakra centers, chakra is of Sanskrit origin and means "circle" or "wheel." They are the subtle energy centers of the body that provide specific energies to support varying physical and spiritual functions within the body. They serve to link those higher vibrational energies to the physical plane of existence. By balancing the energies of a specific chakra, the corresponding physical focus of that chakra can be balanced and healed.

The table on the following page describes the location and energy focus of each primary center. It is important to note that each chakra contains aspects of the other centers. As an example, on Vivienne Simmons' Cosmicwalk web site,[29] she relates how the blockages in the crown chakra can have symptoms in the other Chakras. Some of these symptoms might include an inability to "see" (sight is related to the 5th chakra) our path to spiritual (crown or 7th chakra) enlightenment or a failure to embrace or love (heart or 4th chakra) our spirituality. Laurie Grant also describes this concept in her seminars. Using the ku, lono and aumakua energies as an example, the balance between ku and lono energies in the 4th chakra is equal. As you move lower, the ku gains influence. As you move up, lono is the primary force. The aumakua energies are present in all areas with primary control in the 7th.

29 See http://www.cosmicwalk.com/chakras2.html

The Chakra Centers

Center	Location	Energy Focus
7	Crown of the head	spiritual center, knowingness, pure spirit, higher self, aumakua
6	Center of the head, third eye	Psychic center, perception, creativity, communion with spirit, faithfulness, intellect, knowledge, analysis, trust, brain, eyes, ears, nose, mouth, jaw, middle-self, lono
5	Neck, thyroid	Communication, inspiration, discussion, expression, attitude, truth, throat, middle-self, lono
4	Heart	Unconditional love, affinity, compassion, open heart, release of ego, happiness, service, light, healing, union, family, openness, lungs, middle- and basic-self in equilibrium, balanced lono and ku
3	Solar plexus, just above the navel	Will, will power, discipline, commitment, personality, ego, fear, envy, beauty, pride, digestion, basic self, ku
2	Lower abdomen, ovaries / testes	Emotional, sexual, personal connections, respect for life, relationships, touch, closeness, pleasure, sexual organs, basic self, ku
1	Base of the Spine	Survival, care of the physical self, life, death, struggle, earth, work, inner child, possession, basic self, ku

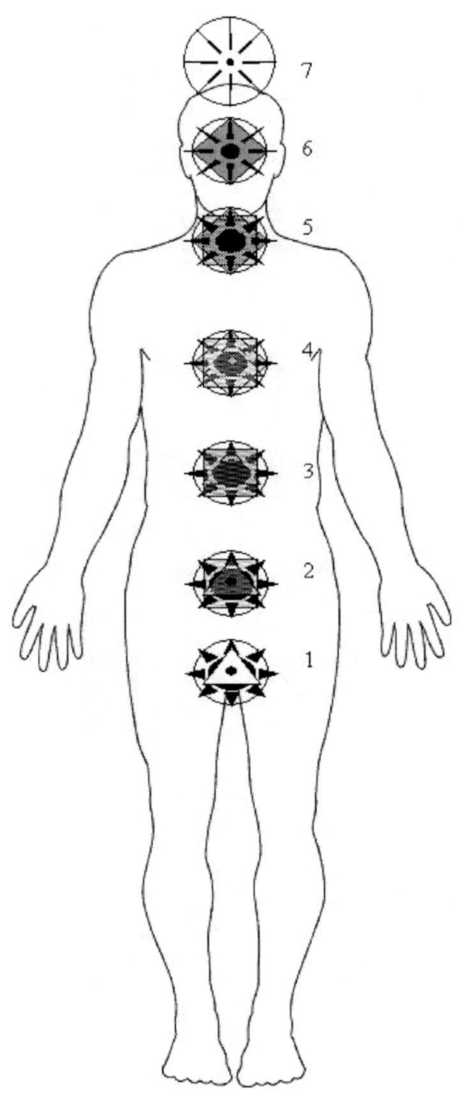

The Chakras

Chapter 5: The Healing Process

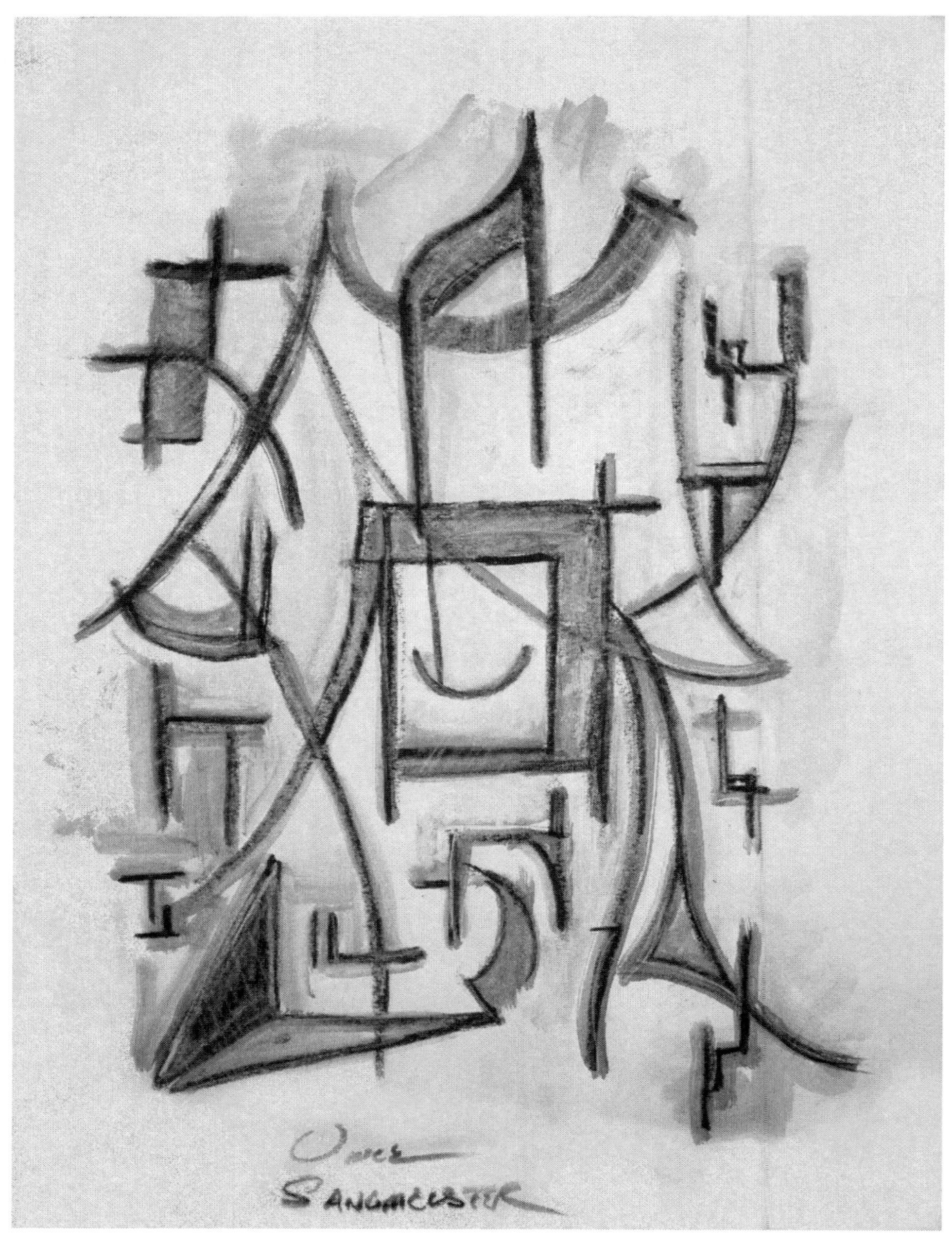

"The Attempt (to Heal)"

There are many bridges under construction. How do we put the pieces together for ourselves?

...as the problem establishes itself in one part, every other part...establishes a new equilibrium (comfort zone) that depends on some of us staying sick! When we begin to induce real improvement...we often see a temporary improvement that does not last until the next treatment. This is why real methods of correction have to be repeated until the entire system has achieved a healthy new equilibrium.

(Dr. Gerald Senogles, licensed Acupuncturist from the "To Your Health" column of Aikido Today magazine #90, Vol. 17, No. 6 – Nov/Dec '03)

In doing healing sessions on clients, I have had many clients relate stories of

- instant healing,
- meeting with God,
- communicating with loved ones who have passed,
- immediate relief or release from a concern, and
- understanding their life's purpose.

A common thread can be seen in many of these experiences: We are not out there, all alone...God does exist!

Some people have reported "instant" healing after working with me. However, several others have required repeat sessions to get to the "root cause" of their "disease." Although healing times are as individual as the clients themselves, there are some common elements that are needed for the healing to take place.

In this chapter, you will find out about the:

- role of faith in healing
- key elements that must be present for healing to occur:
  - Intent
  - Grounding

Questions answered for me in this chapter include:

- How does one heal?
- Why does one heal?

Faith and Healing

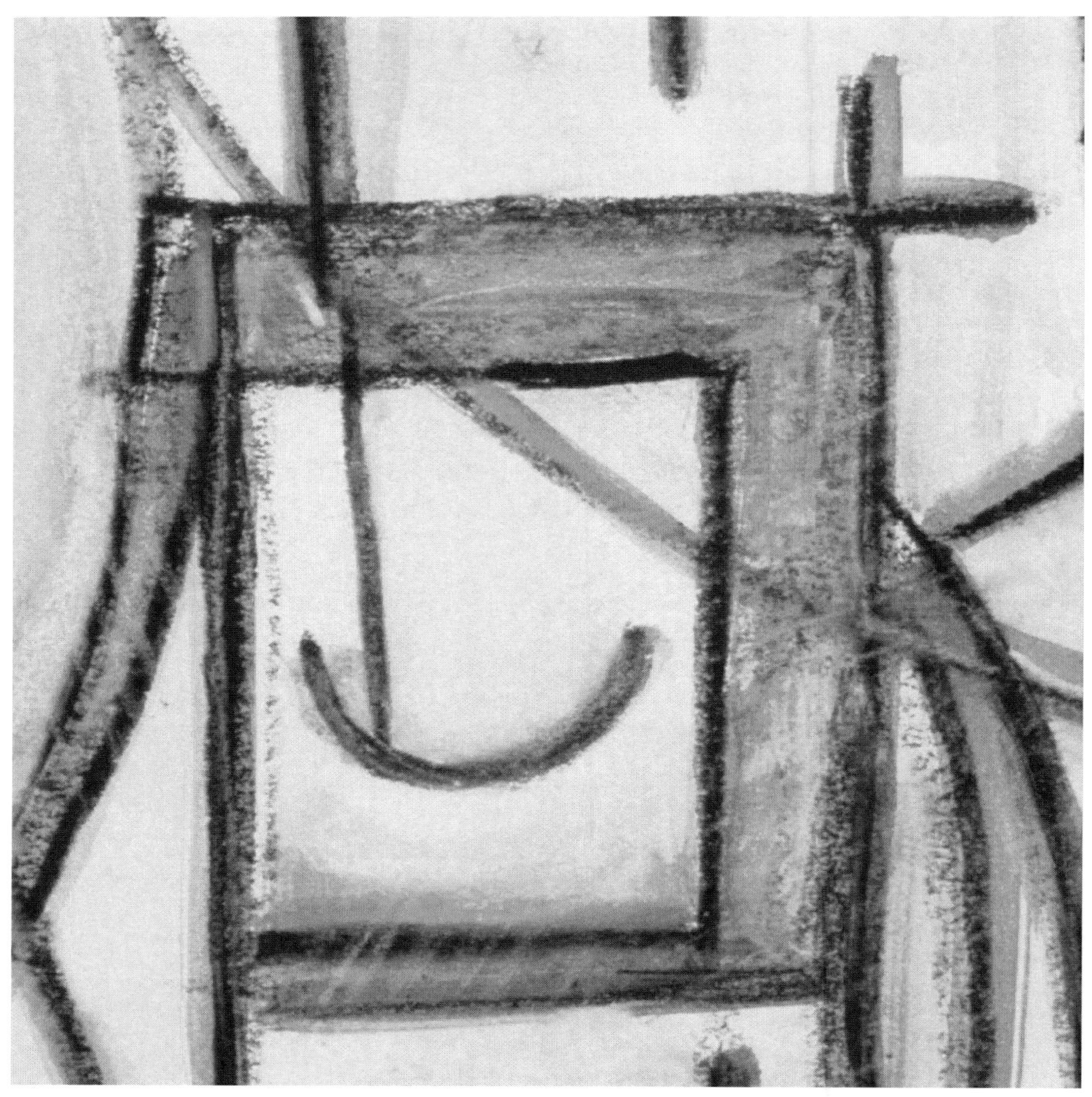

"The Attempt (To Heal)" (detail)

Smile!

Why do some people heal faster than others do?

Why do some injuries and illnesses heal faster?

Healing and the speed at which it happens has very little to do with physio-mechanical (medicine, therapy, etc.) processes. These processes are important and useful in the healing process to change the illness pattern as described by Dr. Senogles at the beginning of this chapter. However, these processes are not the primary requirement for healing to take place.

The key to healing is faith.

Faith knows something is true. When you know, really know, the root cause of an illness or injury, you will heal quickly.

Let us try an experiment to emphasize the ability of the mind to make things so. This is a Feldenkrais® technique that many teachers use.

Stand with your feet about shoulder width apart. Raise one arm and point the index finger at a point in front of you. Now, slowly turn your upper torso, twisting at the waist, in the direction of the arm you raised (turn to the right if your raised your right arm and left for the left arm.) Turn as far as you can without moving your feet. Note where your finger is pointing when you have rotated as far as you can. Return to facing forward.

Now close your eyes and visualize the location where your finger pointed at your maximum rotation. Then visualize a location beyond where your finger pointed. Pick a spot at least 10% farther beyond your current maximum rotation. When visualizing this new location, see yourself easily and effortlessly rotating to this new spot. Truly know that you can do this. Maintain this visualization process until there are no doubts in your mind that you can do this. Have faith that it will happen.

With your eyes still closed and your feet shoulder width apart, raise the same arm and begin to rotate. Rotate like before, as far as you can, without moving your feet. When you have reached your maximum rotation, open your eyes.

I have done and seen this technique done hundreds of times. In nearly all occasions, the person's ability to rotate 10% farther and more has happened easily and effortlessly.

Although a simple example, it demonstrates the mind's ability to influence the body.

Earlier, we talked about people with multiple personalities exhibiting illness in one personality and not in another. This is vivid example of how our state of mind, what we know or what we have faith in, can manifest in our physical consciousness.

Healing the body, mind and soul can be accomplished by having faith and truly believing that the healing will take place. This does not mean necessarily that the healing will take place immediately. There may still be lessons (yours or someone else's) that the illness or injury will facilitate. By acknowledging that you have been offered this situation as a learning experience, believing that you are open to the lessons provided and knowing that you will heal, you have created the conduit to the Divine that will allow the healing to take place.

A highly effective technique for healing can be found in Shamanic practices. Dr. Wesselman does a masterful job in introducing this technique in his book *The Journey to the Sacred Garden: A Guide to Traveling in the Spiritual Realms.*[30] In this book, Dr. Wesselman outlines how one can journey to a special healing place where one can "garden" and change or heal the environment in the Shamanic realm. He then relates how any changes that are made in the Shamanic realm will eventually manifest in the ordinary conscious realm. I have journeyed to my garden on numerous occasions and found it fascinating how the simple act of planting a tree or sweeping the walk in the Shamanic realm can help me become more nurturing or "clean up" my ordinary consciousness.

Healing and enlightenment are like opening a walnut or a flower. If you try to force the walnut or flower open at the wrong time, it is nearly impossible or could cause so much damage that it could never grow to maturity. When the nut is ripe, it easily and gladly opens. When the flower matures, its beauty is revealed.

In healing, the same rules apply. You cannot force someone to heal when he or she has not recognized his or her lesson. Healing without this realization will only deal with the symptom. It is quite possible that the illness will reappear or another illness will manifest to help someone learn the lesson.

It would be against free will for the healer to try to "force" healing on someone. The Divine offers us this energy to heal freely without expectations. We have the free will to use this energy or not. It is up to us. Exercising our free will is taking responsibility for our actions and, consequently, the outcomes. Recognizing our free will helps us to get out of the "victim" mentality. It changes the participant from a "victim" who has had something done to him or her, to a willing participant who made a decision and is accepting of the consequences.

---

30 Dr. Wesselman discusses the healing garden in his book, *The Journey to the Sacred Garden: A Guide to Traveling in the Spiritual Realms*, published by Hay House, Inc., ISBN 1401901115.

As with physical healing, spiritual growth cannot be forced on a person. Unfortunately, the principles of Aikido are not widely practiced. When spirituality is pushed, the person pushes back. It is human nature. There are far too many people in our world trying to force their view of spirituality on us.

You can only show people the door to spirituality and Oneness. They need to initiate crossing the threshold.

Intent

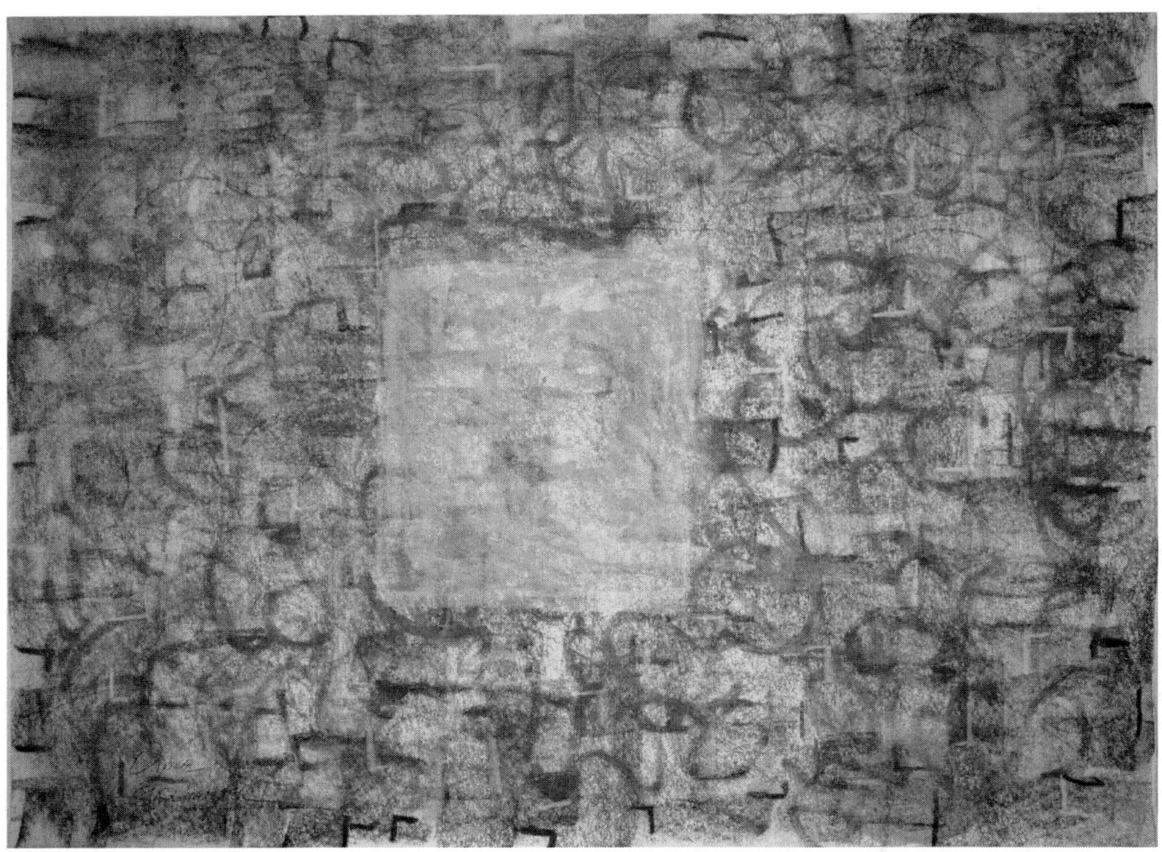

"Centered White"

The chaos surrounds us...as we focus our intention on the goal of Oneness, the white light begins to appear.

It is often hard for us to take that step across the threshold back into Oneness with the Divine Source...especially if we know that it is going to be a big step! One of the things that can help steer us in the right direction is focusing our intention.

Intention is a very important tool that helps a Shaman healer receive information about a client. It is necessary to establish the proper frame of reference that outlines the intention. By establishing the thoughts, feelings and emotions associated with the objective, the Shaman healer is entraining the conscious mind to a vibrational level that will allow the reception and comprehension of the information provided. This same concept applies to the client. The Shaman healer will encourage the client to focus on the situation in order to be receptive to the energy and the messages carried by the energy.

In setting the stage for healing to take place, the Shaman healer will help the client to address the lesson to be learned. The healer will then begin to focus the appropriate energy to support the client's healing efforts. During the session, the healer is always open to the differences in energy flow in each area of the client's body and supporting energy field. This sensitivity allows for an understanding of the needs of the client. If a difference or imbalance is found, the healer will set his or her intention on facilitating the integration of the appropriate energy (at the most beneficial level) into the area. In many cases, the healer will place their hands on corresponding areas of the body (chakra center, strong/healthy area, etc.) and focus on both hands in order to help the client support the positive energy flow.

By focusing on both hands at the same time, the healer is bringing into agreement the right and left, male and female, yin and yang – in other words, the duality of existence. This allows the healer to concentrate the energies and call on the Divine Source to come into Oneness with the client and support the healing.

A small prayer is then said asking that the area heal instantly, if it is for the client's greatest good. The last statement is of utmost importance. It is possible that the client has additional learning to be facilitated by this ailment and, therefore, it is necessary for the situation to continue. Even in these cases, there is healing. This can be as simple as the person recognizing the lesson to be learned or receiving information that puts them on the path to the learning.

The Universe is constantly supplying us with information. Sometimes we receive the information without intention and rationalize it as intuition or the "little voice inside my head." These are instances when your unconscious understands your objective or the information you require – and then extracts the information from the universal stream of knowledge. When a healer is attempting to gather information on the client's behalf in order to facilitate a healing, the healer needs to ensure that his or her conscious self is able to understand and articulate this information to the client. By establishing intention and by fixing consciousness on the vibrational level of the information to be received, the healer tunes his normal, conscious vibrational level to the level of the Universe. By doing this, the Universe supplies information to the lower self or ku. In turn, the ku is able to receive the information, understand that the information is important and pass the information to the middle-self or lono or mind. The lono is then able to interpret and understand the information and pass it onto the client.

Not tuning into the vibration of the information would be like opening a volume of an encyclopedia, turning randomly to a page, reading two lines, then being expected to understand what you read and what the subject of the entry was. This makes misinterpretation of the data quite likely. By fixing intention, thoughts, feelings and emotions on the objective, the healer knows that he is opening the "A" volume of the encyclopedia and is reading two lines from the "Aardvark" entry. The knowledge can then be put into context. This offers the healer a better chance of interpreting the data correctly and the client a higher probability of accepting and using the information to heal.

Intention also helps the Shaman use the information and energy to the benefit of all the parties involved in a situation. The energy with which the Shaman is working can be likened to electricity. Electricity can be used to benefit humanity through light, heat, transportation, information exchange, etc. The very same electricity that powers your house can kill if not handled properly or when used to destroy, such as in the execution of a condemned inmate. It is the intention of the person using the electricity as to how it will serve. The electricity does not judge. It simply **is**.

The same is true for the Shaman. This Divine energy can be used for benefit or detriment. This is why it is imperative that the Shaman uses this energy with a beneficial intention. The outcome depends on the intention of the Shaman. Intention also helps both the Shaman healer and the client to imagine the outcome. The intention leads to the image, that leads to the faith, that is empowered by the energy to manifest.

Grounding

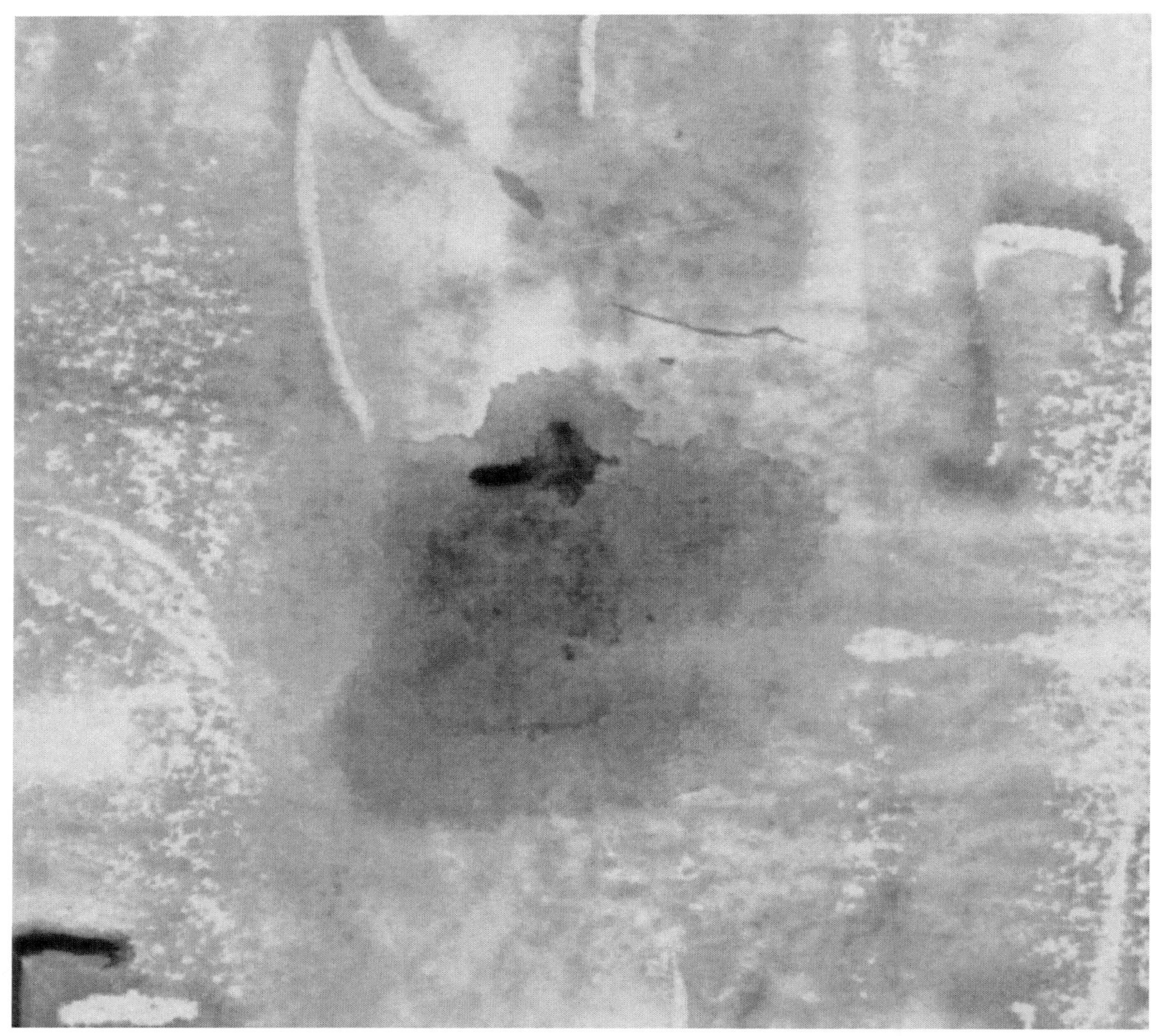

***"Filtered and Refocused"* (detail)**

Grounding enables you to find that central point that can be used as an anchor.

Besides focusing your intention for the purpose of directing the necessary energy, the healer (or heal-ee) must also ground the energy being transmitted or received.

This is very important for the health and well-being of the Shaman and the client. When the Shaman grounds the spiritual energies, he does not simply run the spiritual energy down into the earth like a lightening rod. The grounding is accomplished by balancing the spiritual energies with the corresponding earth energies. I learned from Laurie Grant of a Kahuna saying, "You can only bring down as much energy as you bring up." This concept teaches the equality of heaven and earth energies.

Grounding is accomplished by focusing your intention to act as a bridge between the spiritual and earth energies with which you are interacting. In essence, you are helping to rejoin the duality of heaven and earth through this act and rebuilding Oneness. Your intention is to allow the spiritual energy to pass through you like water in a stream flowing over rocks. You are "wetting" and spiritually charging each of your Chakra centers by its passing, taking only what is needed. This energy is then offered to the Earth Spirit as a gift. Some people see this energy anchored at the center of the earth as providing a feeling of safety and security.

Similarly, you allow the earth energies to rise up through each Chakra, reconnecting you with the earth and its healing energy. Additionally, these energies are blending and becoming one within you...a balancing of Heaven and Earth. These energies are then offered to the spiritual realms as an offering of gratitude.

By not grounding, you become like an over-charged or un-used battery. In the over-charged battery analogy, the energy (spiritual or earth) builds in your body and begins to overload your Chakras. This causes an imbalance and can lead to unwanted issues like a feeling of buzzing and not being able to stop. Conversely, in the un-used battery example, the energy becomes stagnant and begins to lose potency. The un-used battery eventually becomes difficult to "re-charge."

Because the earth and spiritual energies are equally important, the decision on which to connect with first is up to you. It is important to know your own body and which type of energy you most resonate. People and animals tend to have a natural affinity to energy. Some are more grounded and more closely aligned with earth energy. Others are operating at a higher frequency and are more aligned with spiritual energy.

In the cases of animals, former students of mine have told me that their dog would not sit still for a treatment or their cat seemed to be "spooked" after a session. I believe that an excess of either earth or spiritual energy causes this. In these situations, it may help to ground the "clients" (people, dogs, cats, etc.) prior to the session.

For example, the dog who would not sit still might be more open to the energy if he were first fully grounded with his natural earth energy. This action would place the dog into a calm, relaxed state prior to introducing the spiritual energy. For animals more aligned with spiritual energy, you could start with introducing the spiritual energy then moving to the earth energy.

Types of Healing Treatments

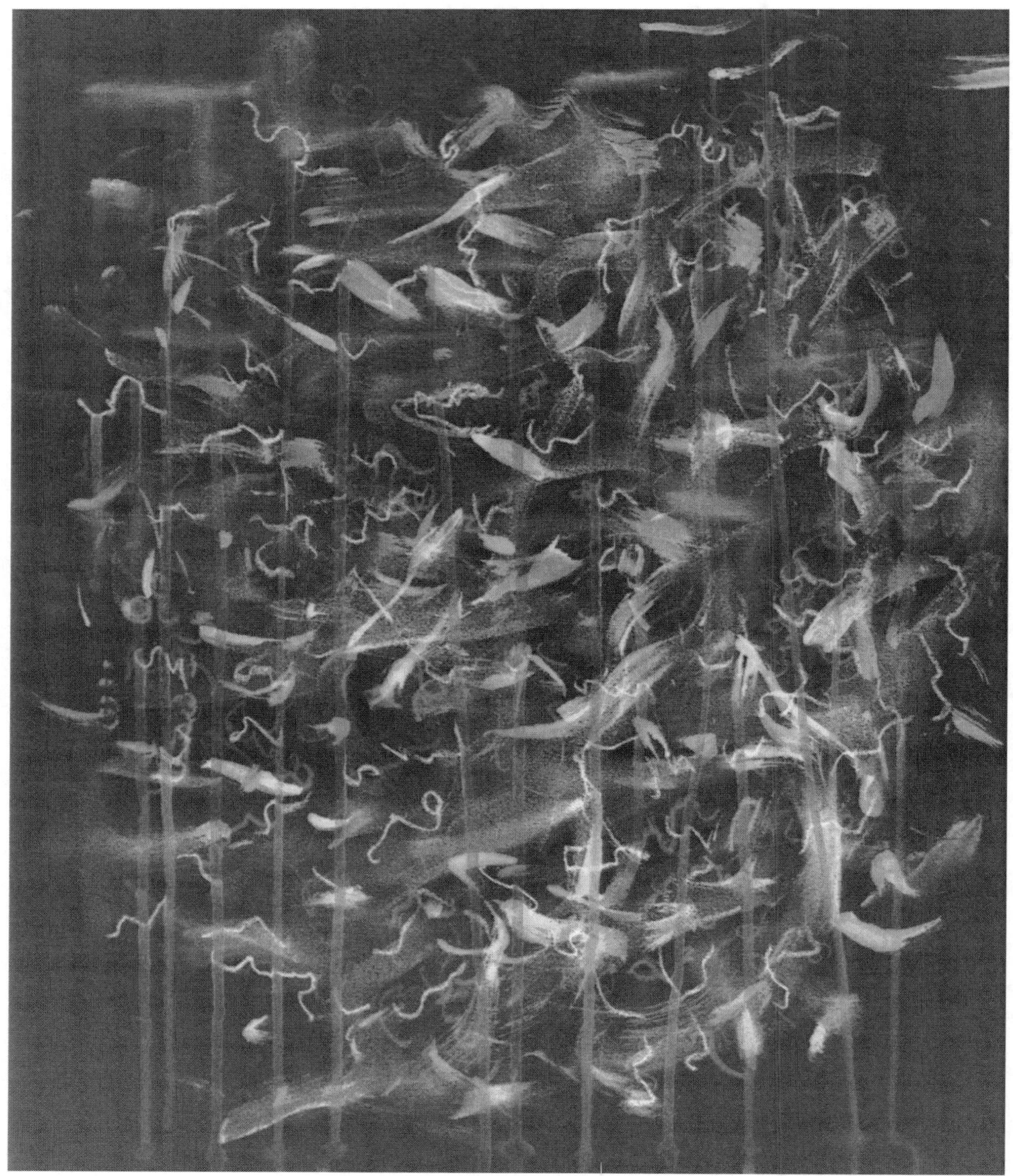

"Active" (negative image, detail)

There are always under currents of energy behind the myriad of paths back to Oneness.

There are many different tools that a Shaman has available to treat a client. These include face-to-face and remote treatments that can focus on an individual, groups, objects or the whole world.

The most common treatments are done in person. These sessions are normally conducted with the client sitting or lying on a table or the floor. The choice of position is predicated on the comfort of the client and/or the needs of the Shaman.

During remote treatments, the healer may either:

- enter a Shamanic state and "journey" to the client, or
- ask the client's spirit or being do the "traveling."

Once the connection is made, the remote treatment is conducted in a similar fashion to the face-to-face treatment described earlier.

If the Shaman journeys, two options are available:

- work on the client's spirit, or
- work directly on the client's physical body.

This decision is totally up to the Shaman, depending on the state of the client. If the Shaman is considering having the client's spirit travel, the risk of that spirit permanently leaving the physical body needs to be examined. One risk might be if the client is in a coma and it is unclear whether he or she wishes to leave this existence at this time. If the Shaman were to request the presence of the spirit, the client's decision might be affected.

For worldwide treatment, energy is directed to the affected geographic area. The energy is offered freely for the benefit of anyone and/or anything in need.

It is important to note that the healing energies must never be forced on anyone or anything. They are offered as a gift to be accepted or rejected without judgment.

This type of alternative treatment is just that – an alternative. Many people are quick to discount the knowledge and training of doctors and therapists trained through our educational institutions. What is being offered in this book is a different way of looking at illness and how clients are treated. We also need to honor the skill of our medical professionals. When you are bleeding severely, go to the hospital! When you want to find out what lesson you need to learn from life, seek the Shaman or alternative practitioner. Shamanic treatments are not a substitute for the care of traditional and/or holistic medical professionals.

Chapter 6: Origin of Hawaiian Beliefs

"CD1 Cut1" (detail)

Bali Hai is calling...Many cultures know that their present location is a result of the travels of long-lost ancestors. That connection forms the way that they view their world.

When a man is singing and cannot lift his voice, and another comes and sings with him, another who can lift his voice, the first will be able to lift his voice too. That is the secret of the bond between spirits.
- Hasidic saying

Throughout this journey, I have fought an internal battle between the left and right sides of my brain. My intuition (or right side of the brain) is telling me that I was learning the truth, while my logic circuit (or left side of the brain) craved supporting facts or words to explain the unexplainable. The following is my attempt to "lift my voice" and apply facts in order to make historical connections between all that has been discussed.

In this chapter, you will find out about common themes that link the Hawaiian beliefs to the ancient world.

Questions answered for me in this chapter include:

- Where did the Hawaiians originate?
- How can an isolated race develop Spiritual beliefs so much like those found in the ancient world?

Common Ties

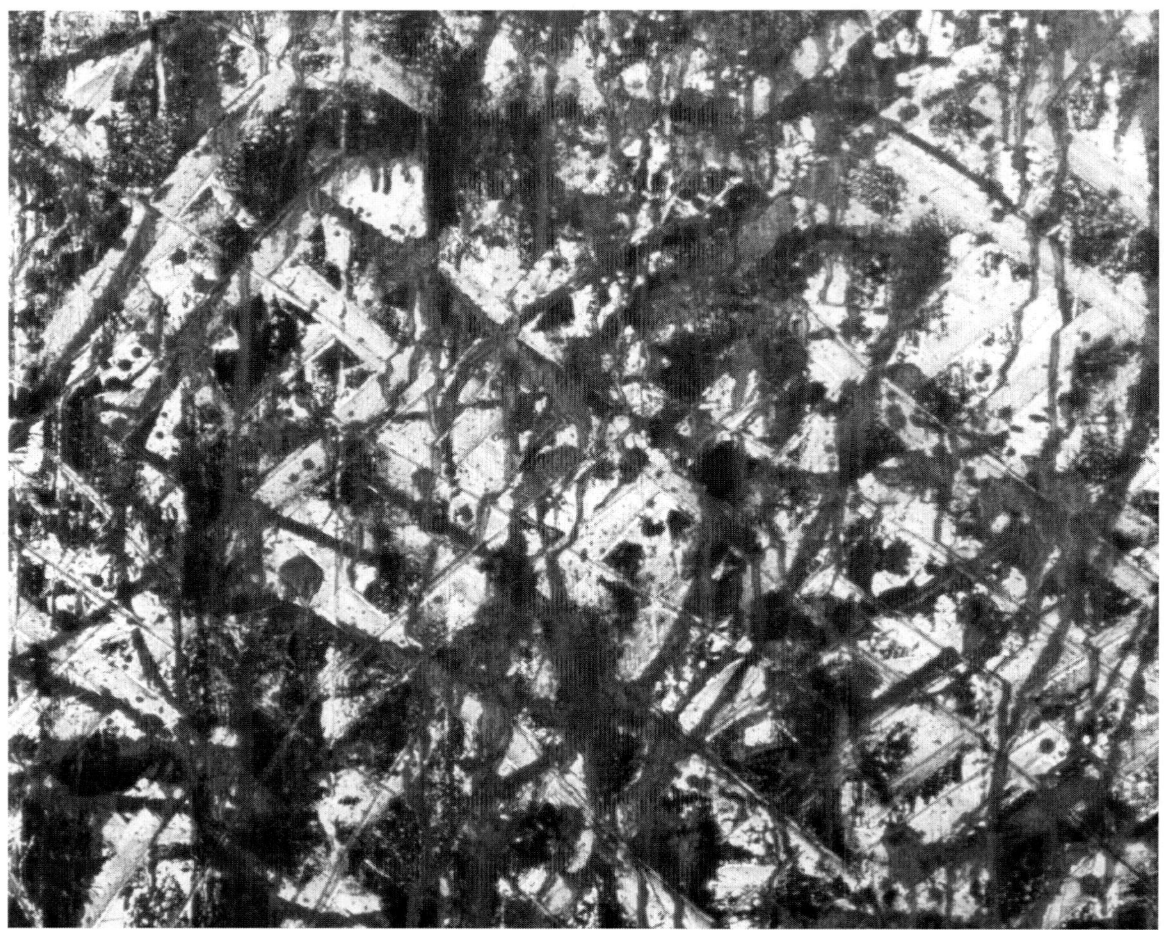

"Blue Agony Resurrection" (detail)

We are all connected. As we change our focus, the lines of connection become clearer and continue to grow...the energy connections increase.

As we have seen, there are similarities between many of the world's religions and a possibility that there is an underlying, common history to these beliefs. It also appears that the Hawaiians and Polynesians share these common understandings. How did races of people so isolated develop these beliefs? Is it possible that the Hawaiians and Polynesians owe their linage to the people of the ancient world, specifically Africa?

As an example of a tie between Hawaii and Africa, common names for stars, creation stories and family lineages were discovered during a meeting between a Hawaiian elder and an African elder.[31] The most interesting revelation from this meeting centered on their common ancestor.

Upon meeting each other, the elders recited their ancestral lineages so that they could understand "who the person is." Such practice is common in indigenous cultures. While the African elder spoke, the Hawaiian elder realized that their respective lineages were the same! In particular, the African related the story of a great warrior that had set sail from his homeland but had never returned. It is customary in seafaring societies that the explorer return or send a representative back to their point of origin so that the lines of communication can be maintained. The great African warrior's name was Maui, one of the greatest heroes of Hawaiian history. According to the African elder, Maui, his ancestor, had set sail and had never been heard from again.

The Hawaiian elder then proceeded to relate his ancestral lineage and complete the story of Maui's exploits, thereby completing the voyage of Maui that began so many centuries before.

According to historian Abraham Fornander,[32] the Hawaiians migrated from an original, ancient people who probably lived in the area of Persia. He documents that he can confidently place the Hawaiian ancestors in ancient India with the Vedic Arian, Dravidians, Arab Cushites and African Chaldeans. He speculates that there are further linkages taking the lineage into pre-Deluvian Africa.

---

31 This information was derived from a report on the Worldwide Indigenous Science Network website (http://www.wisn.org) and through meetings with the Hawaiian elder mentioned.

32 See *An Account of The Polynesian Race its Origin and Migrations and Ancient History of the Hawaiian People to the Times of Kamehameha I* by Abraham Fornander, published by Charles E. Tuttle Company, ISBN 0804800022.

There is more evidence. Many of the ancient Hawaiian stories mirror or match ancient Hebrew/Bible stories including:

- Creation,
- Adam and Eve,
- Number of generations between the first man and the "flood,"
- Noah (Nuu in Hawaiian),
- Number of generations between Noah (the savior of man) and the "next" Noah whose story mirrors the Biblical Abraham,
- Views of reality (like the similarities between the Hawaiian and Kabbalistic views discussed earlier), and
- Cities of refuge, like:
    - The Hawaiian Places of Refuge – Pu'uhonua o Honaunau – on the Big Island of Hawaii, that would accept, welcome and provide safe haven for all who reached its walls,
    - Those described in the Bible (Numbers 35:6), and
    - The temple of Ceres at Hermione that was a city of refuge in ancient Greece.

One of the most significant parallels is the name of the Hawaiian Supreme Being or "the primordial cosmic force of Creation"[33] known as Teawe or Keawe. In the Hawaiian language, this name would be pronounced tay-yah-vay or kay-yah-vay. Hawaiian words can be broken down into their components to determine the underlying or secret meaning. If we apply this technique to Keawe, one possible translation is as follows:

kea or kaya or kela – the absolute, supreme

we or ve – source, origin

or, as a phrase, the Supreme Source.

In Hebrew, YHWH, pronounced ya-way, is the Supreme Being.

---

33 This definition/translation of Keawe is from Julius Scammon Rodman's book, *The Kahuna Sorcerers of Hawaii, Past and Present*, published in 1979 by Exposition Press, Inc. ISBN: 0682491969.

Furthermore, there are stories of a lost tribe of Israel. I think that it is possible that this story is a re-telling of an older story of the migration of an ancient race from the area of North Africa to the east. The similarities in terms of a Supreme Being and the other common stories point to the possibility that the Hebrews and Hawaiians originated from an even older, original race.

Additionally, Fornander makes the observation that one key to telling the antiquity of a race is by the complexity of the culture's numbering system. He notes that the Hawaiians, along with the ancient Vedics and Cushites, have the number four as their base unit versus our number ten. From this, he further hypothesizes that these cultures are branches of a much older culture.

Further evidence of the antiquity of the original Hawaiian race can be found in the Hawaiian creation story, the Kumulipo. The story, normally recited as a chant, talks of the creation of many plants and animals, some of which do not exist or never have existed in Polynesia. This fact seems to indicate that these histories originate from a different place where these plants and animals did/do exist. Of special interest is that the Kumulipo does <u>not</u> mention palm trees or coconuts. This seems to be an extreme oversight given the preponderance of this plant throughout Polynesia.

Supplementary information on the antiquity of the Kumulipo comes from the Bishop Museum in Hawaii, the chief source of information on ancient Hawaii and Polynesian culture. The Museum has done an analysis comparing the Hawaiian Kumulipo to the scientific taxonomy of the origins of life on this planet.[34] This study found numerous similarities between the progression of life according to the Kumulipo and the evidence found by archeologists in the fossil records.

The report mapped The First Age (Wa Akahi) as described in the Kumulipo to the Cambrian period, 570 million years ago, when the first sea life developed; including marine invertebrates and shell-bearing animals.

In many cases where the Kumulipo and scientific versions of creation differed, the Kumulipo validated that a specific life form appeared prior to the fossil record.

For example, the Kumulipo tells that pigs appeared as the first mammals after the first reptiles during the "Time of the Night Diggers" (Ka Wa Elima) about 180 million years ago. Science also indicates that the first mammals appeared during this time.

34 See the Bishop Museum web site for additional information (http://explorers.bishopmuseum.org).

A similar pattern is found with birds. The Kumulipo places the first birds on earth approximately 345 million years ago during "The Time of the Winged Creatures" (Ka Wa Ekolu) after the appearance of bony fishes. Science shows that the ancestors to dinosaurs appear during this time. It is interesting that science now believes that present day birds are distant relatives of the dinosaurs.

Although not scientifically proven, it is possible that archeologists have not found the oldest fossil samples to date and that the species like pigs appeared earlier than currently believed. Our science has done and continues to do a stellar job at explaining and researching the world's history. It, however, approaches history with a very tactile view. If a scientist can touch an artifact, then he is free to hypothesize on the origins, culture, lifestyle and thoughts of the originator of the artifact. Although this is a safe way to view the world, it leads to science with "blinders." Many of the ideas that I have been offered do not fit the current "blind" science. You cannot touch Divine Source Energy. At this time, you cannot measure it. There was a time, not long ago, when one could not measure energy coming from stars millions of light-years away. Did that energy not exist prior to the time when our technology "discovered" it?

Egyptian Connection

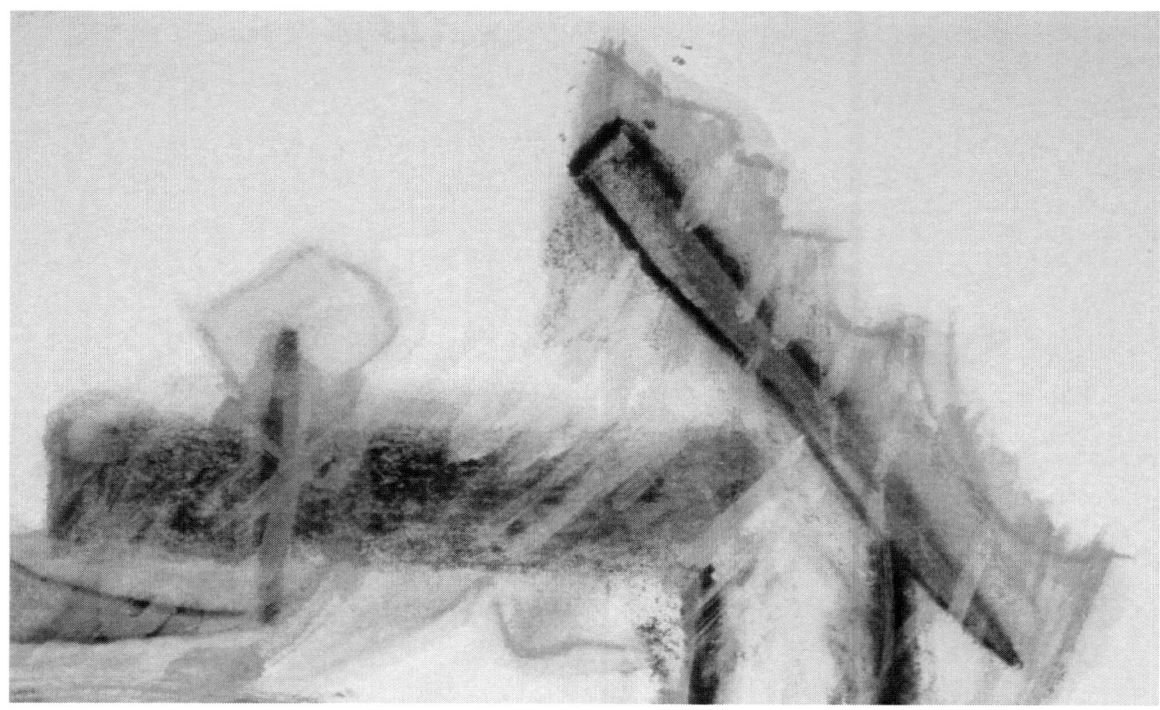

"Coeur" (detail)

The ability of a structure to store or transmit energy was a significant aspect of the designs of Egyptian builders. When you "build" or co-create, you can infuse your creation with Divine Source Energy.

When I began my studies of Shamanism, I learned about the 26,000-year cycle of our solar system as it transits the Milky Way Galaxy. I found out that, like night and day, the cycle has 13,000 years of darkness and 13,000 of illumination. Many put great emphasis on the night and day, light and dark, aspects of this cycle. It is believed that there is an increase in consciousness during the "light" phase of the cycle.

Since we now re-enter one of these "light" phases, this theory indicates that the last time when consciousness was at its highest was approximately 13,000 years ago – in an ancient time.

It is believed that the Hawaiian healing techniques originated in one of the most ancient cultures that we know of – the Egyptian culture. This seems to track with historian Abraham Fornander's investigation of the origins of the Hawaiian people and ancient stories from African and Hawaiian elders placing their original race in the middle-east and Africa. Further, the mystical experiences of Dr. Hank Wesselman and Laurie Grant, among others, have indicated the possibility of an Egyptian / Hawaiian connection.

As I said earlier, there are theories that this migration to Hawaii happened approximately 12,500 years ago. I was intrigued by the possibility that evidence might exist of a migration of peoples from Egypt to Hawaii, a migration that could have brought the ancient teachings and consciousness that existed at the close of the last "light" cycle.

I found several interesting articles that provide potential proof that ancient Egyptians traveled widely, reaching at least as far as Australia.

Researcher Paul White[35] describes extremely ancient Egyptian hieroglyphs that were discovered in a National Park in New South Wales, Australia. The hieroglyphs tell the tale of early Egyptian explorers, injured and stranded, in ancient Australia.

According to White, Egyptologist Ray Johnson translated the characters. Johnson indicated that the hieroglyphs stemmed from the Egyptian Third Dynasty. The hieroglyphs document the fate of the leader of the expedition, "Lord Djes-eb." Apparently, the expedition was shipwrecked in a land, which they described as a "wretched place."

Through the hieroglyphs, which record the name of "RA-JEDEF" as reigning King of the Upper and Lower Nile and son of "KHUFU" who, in turn, is son of the King "SNEFERU," the date of the expedition is estimated between 2748 and 1779 B.C. This period is just after the reign of King Khufu, who is also known as "Cheops," the reputed builder of the Great Pyramid. Lord Djes-eb may have actually been one of the sons of the Pharaoh Ra Djedef, who reigned after Khufu.

---

35 A complete account of these hieroglyphs, see http://www.crystalinks.com/egyptaustralia.html and http://www.kachina.net/~alunajoy/articles.html.

Some theorists put forward that Australia is the fabled "lost motherland" in the Pacific of the Sumerians, Mayans, Hawaiians and other cultures. It seems fairly certain that the maritime civilizations of antiquity were quite capable of extensive ocean voyages.

There is evidence that early Egyptians were just this type of civilization. In the 1950's, a 4,500-year old, 100-foot, ocean-going vessel was excavated in the vicinity of the Great Pyramid. In 1991, several even older boats were found buried in the desert at Abydos in Upper Egypt. According to the Cairo Times in 1982, archaeologists working at Fayum, near the Siwa Oasis uncovered fossils of kangaroos and other Australian marsupials. In addition, there is a strange set of golden boomerangs discovered by Professor Carter in the tomb of Tutankhamen in 1922.

This information offers supporting evidence that the Egyptians traveled between Egypt and Australia. There is additional data supporting the sea-faring nature of the early Egyptians.

This theory is offered in Edo Nyland's[36] discussion of the "People of the Sea." It is thought that the People of the Sea were a people of the Saharan area prior to the desertification of Northern Africa. The Saharans are thought to have perfected boat-building, sailing and star navigation. Their livelihood was totally dependent on the sea. Nyland writes that the People of the Sea:

> "...may have started their experimentation on the ocean as early as 40,000 years ago and had learned that the sea could provide a reliable food supply at all times of the year and as a result had developed highly advanced, sea-food harvesting methods. When the central Sahara became unlivable because of fast advancing desertification which forced them to flee to the coast, the Sea Peoples were ready and available to ferry the displaced tribes and their livestock north to Europe."

In support of Nyland's assertion of a pre-historic race influencing the early Egyptians, the original view by the Egyptian people of their gods was not that of supreme beings looking down from on high. Ancient Egyptians viewed their gods as men who could live and die with all the frailties of humans (anger, greed, sadness, etc.) There were even cemeteries set aside specifically for these gods. Why would a group place god-like status on individuals who were most certainly human?

In times of superstition, the simplest act could be viewed as "magic." Things like healing skills or the ability to harness the wind for sailing or find fish by connecting with the fish spirits, would be viewed as a god-like in ancient times. These god-men could be the Saharans Nyland describes.

I find that Nyland's description of this race could be directly applied to the Polynesians and Hawaiians, specifically his description of a highly advanced sea-faring

---

36 See *Linguistic Archaeology* by Edo Nyland, published by Trafford, Victoria, B.C. Available at http://www.trafford.com/robots/01-0069.html.

race that harvested the ocean. For centuries, the Hawaiians used, and still use, man-made fish ponds to store their catches for future consumption.

One argument immediately comes to mind concerning the Saharans: Why would have a race who lived by harvesting the oceans, stopped fishing?

Logic dictates that if the race continued to fish and thrive throughout pre-history and into known history, they would have left archeological traces of their civilization. I do not believe that the Saharans continued to fish the Mediterranean, due a climatic by-product of the melting of the ice cap at the end of the last ice age.

This event is called the Younger Dryas, which happened approximately 11,500 to 13,000 years ago. During a 1,000-year period, the climate of at least the North Atlantic area, and potentially globally, went through a "cold snap" when the Gulf Stream was shut down due to a fresh water cap from the melting glaciers. Europe was especially hard hit by the Younger Dryas. This type of climatic upheaval would have made finding and catching fish difficult. The colder temperatures of the normal fishing areas coupled with a cap of fresh water would have forced the fish population to find more hospitable conditions or die.

But where did the people go?

Approximately 12,000-years ago, the Natufian culture began to purposely cultivate cereal grains in the Mediterranean area. They were some of the first people to do this. Up until this time, the people foraged for cereals. It seems possible that a people whose main food source, fish, had vanished would turn to agriculture as a viable alternative to starvation.

Now that we have established that the Egyptians and their potential ancestors, the Saharans, were seafarers, we will now look at additional links between the Hawaiians, the Saharans and the Egyptians.

Linguistic Connections

"Interstice II"

Although we may not have the knowledge to understand what is being said, a few of the words sound familiar. They connect us and identify an underlying pattern.

In Genesis 11:1, it is stated: “The whole earth was of one lip and of one speech.” This is commonly interpreted to mean that all peoples on earth spoke the same language and could communicate freely. This language could be called the Universal language. According to a controversial theory brought forth by Edo Nyland in his book *Linguistic Archeology,*[37] the world’s languages were “invented” from an ancient language spoken by the people of North Africa and the Near East, who fled this land at the close of the last Ice Age, as this area became the Sahara Desert. Nyland theorizes that this language, which he calls Saharan, is still spoken in an altered form by the Dravidians of India, the Basques of Euskadi and the Ainu of Japan. Nyland considers Basque to most closely resemble ancient Saharan.

Genesis 11:7 states: "Come, let us go down and confuse their language so that they cannot understand one another's speech." This was done because the “common man” was developing an understanding of his direct connection with the Divine. This understanding would have undermined the status of the “priests” or “leaders.” It is possible that the clergy of Judaism spent an enormous and long-sustained effort to bring about this confusion, documenting their actions as a command from God.

In Serge Kahili King’s book *Mastering Your Hidden Self,*[38] he relates a Kahuna belief that, in antiquity, an artificial language was created by those who were initiated into primordial religious practices. This language was to be used to pass on their knowledge. According to the Kahuna, this language is the root of all languages, thereby permitting the spirit of the original knowledge to be carried through all time.

Nyland has evaluated many of the ancient languages, both dead and spoken, using the “short-hand” method where each syllable of a word represents a vowel-consonant-vowel (VCV) combination that is found at the beginning of the original word. In combination, the last vowel in the VCV is the same as the first vowel in the next triad (i.e., VCV^1 - V^1CV^2 - V^2CV^3). Some words began as vowel-vowel (VV).

37 See *Linguistic Archaeology* by Edo Nyland, published by Trafford, Victoria, B.C. Available at http://www.trafford.com/robots/01-0069.html.

38 *Mastering Your Hidden Self* by Serge Kahili King, published by Theosophical Publishing House; (April 1985). ISBN 0835605914.

This technique is best observed through example from Nyland's web site.[39]

"The Basques call their own language Euskera. When analyzed using the VCV/VV method, Euskera is broken down as (* indicates that a vowel was dropped):

eu - us* - *ke - era

and with further refinement:

eu - usa - ake - era

then expanded to complete Basque words:

euki - usaiako - akela - erabildura

In English, these words are translated as:

Euki – to retain/preserve

Usaiako – usual/traditional

Akela – Goddess

Era – usage/speech

or

We preserve the traditional speech of the Goddess"

39 See *Linguistic Archaeology* by Edo Nyland, published by Trafford, Victoria, B.C. Available at http://www.trafford.com/robots/01-0069.html.

Nyland notes that "this would be a logical construction technique within a language. However, this pattern appears to repeat between many languages including Sanskrit, Hebrew, English and Egyptian among others."

Nyland also shows an Egyptian example:

egi - ip* - *t*

then to:

egi - ipu - uto

expanded to full words as:

egin - ipuin - utopia

in English:

egin – to create

ipuin – legend

utopia – utopia

or

They created the legend of utopia.[40]

The tie between Basque and Ainu can be observed through a table found in Mr. Nyland's book. The table provides 117 examples of Basque and Ainu words that are the same or similar, with identical or related meanings. There are a few examples on the next page.

40 Source: *Linguistic Archaeology* by Edo Nyland, published by Trafford, Victoria, B.C. Available at http://www.trafford.com/robots/01-0069.html.

The contents of this table were excerpted from Nyland's book.[41] From a pronunciation standpoint, the Basque "s" is pronounced as a soft "sh" and our sharp "sh" is written as "x."

AINU	***ENGLISH***	***BASQUE***	***ENGLISH***
tontone	to be bald	tontordun	crested / plumed
taspare	to sigh	asparen	to sigh
aske	hand	esku	hand
hera	to limp	herren	cripple
tur	dirt	lur	dirt
mokor	sleep	makar	sleep
tasum	illness	eritasun	illness
araka	illness	arakatu	to be examined
usante	to marry	usantza	tradition
sikupu	to perish	siku	shriveled up
kayo	to cry out	kaio	seagull
kaya	sail	kaiar	very large seagull
ikoro	money	koro	money
erama	to get used to	eramanpen	patience / tolerance

Ainu is considered an isolated language, relatively untouched by outside influences. From the chart, it seems likely that the Basque and Ainu languages have a common ancestry potentially showing a multi-path migration from the drying Sahara region northward into Europe and then to the east into the Japanese island chain.

A tie between Hawaii and this area of the ancient world can be found in the linguistics of the ancient teachings that brought forth at least two of the world's great religions, Judaism and Christianity. During discussions at the 2002 Prophets' Conference in Santa Fe,

---

41 Source: *Linguistic Archaeology* by Edo Nyland, published by Trafford, Victoria, B.C. Available at http://www.trafford.com/robots/01-0069.html.

New Mexico,[42] Shaman and anthropologist Dr. Hank Wesselman stated that the name of the Creator in ancient Hawaiian was IAO. This was of great interest to spiritual researcher Gregg Braden. Braden indicated that he had determined that in the ancient Hebrew writings, all letters of the alphabet were utilized and could be part of anyone's vocabulary except I, A and O. These letters were only used by the priests.

An additional thread of evidence linking the Hawaiians to the Egyptians can be found when analyzing the treatment of the Egyptian kings. The Egyptian kings were thought to be gods who incarnated to serve their people. Upon his death, the king would undergo a secret ceremony that elevated him or her to true god status. This was also the practice of the Hawaiians. When a Hawaiian king died, he was thought to become a god. It was thought that the power of the god was stored in his bones. The bones were placed in the deceased king's heiau or shrine. His godly mana or life force would then be of support to his people for all times.

There was a second part to the Egyptian ceremony that ties into our previous topic of Shamanism. The new king would accompany the deceased king into the temple, or possibly the pyramid, to complete the king-making and, therefore, god-making ceremony. During the ceremony, the new king would undergo a symbolic death when he would accompany the old king through the heavens. During this time, the new king would be blessed by the spirits and he would return to the temple re-born as the god-king. This ceremony bears a striking resemblance to the symbolic death initiation that Shamans go through. During a Shamanic journey, the new Shaman experiences "watching" himself being killed and eaten by a wild animal spirit like a lion or bear. Once the deed is complete, the animal that killed or a different power animal spirit will re-construct the newly initiated Shaman. This re-construction process is viewed as imparting sacred knowledge to the Shaman that will prepare him or her to complete his duty to his community – and align his new body's structure more with the spirit world.

Taking into consideration the data presented above, it seems possible that the ancient Polynesians and Hawaiians were descendants of the ancient Saharans. I find it of extreme significance that two researchers (Fornander and Nyland) – nearly a century apart, through different scientific methods – both traced the Hawaiian culture back to Africa.

---

42 For additional information on the Prophet's Conference and to order a recording of the session to hear this interaction, see the conference web site http://www.greatmystery.org.

Further Migrations

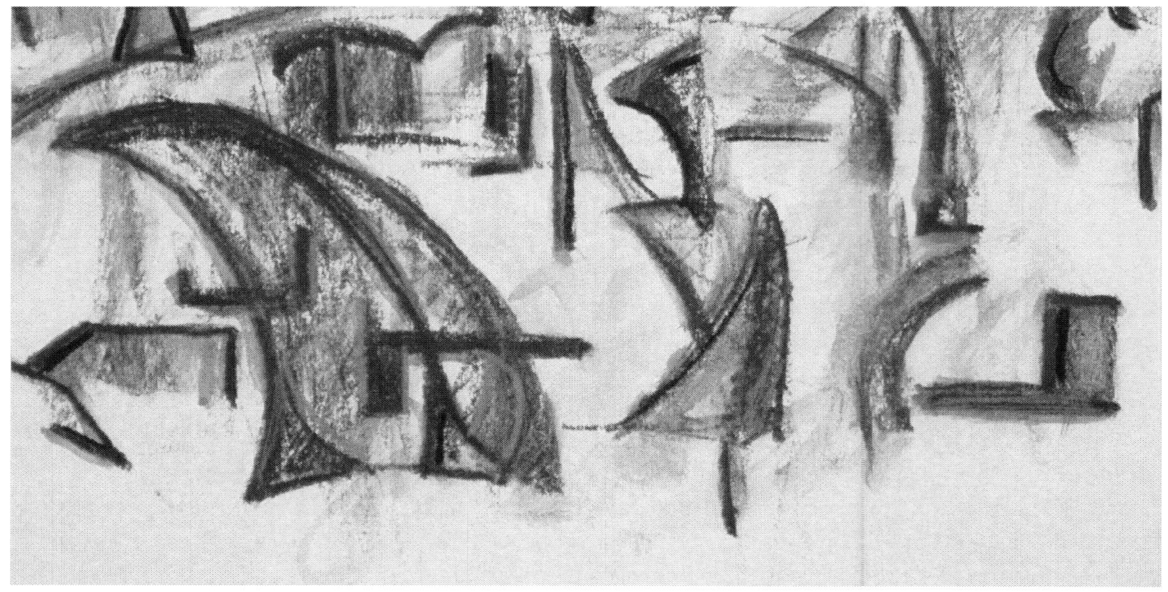

"Fractured Self" (detail)

Even in paradise, the need to explore the path leads to sails moving across the ocean.

Based on my research, I feel there is a strong possibility that the original, sea-going Hawaiians were not content with remaining in one place for long, even after finding the paradise of the Hawaiian Island chain. While doing research on rainbows, a very prominent part of Hawaiian life, I ran across a very curious set of coincidences that provides some interesting connections between the ancient Hawaiians and the Chumash Indians of the central/southern California coast.

I found a fascinating book titled *The Rainbow Bridge* by Audrey Wood.[43] In this book, Wood retells the Chumash creation myth. According to the oral tradition, the tribe came into existence when the goddess Hutash planted seeds on an island called Limuw, which may be a reference to the fabled Lemuria.[44]

Instead of plants, humans grew out of the ground. Unfortunately, the island became crowded and Hutash created a rainbow linking the island with the mainland. Many humans walked over the bridge and populated the new land. As the people were crossing the bridge, a storm appeared and several of the humans fell into the ocean, where they were turned into dolphins.

I believe that this "myth" is the story of the migration of the Hawaiians to the west coast of the Americas.

After further researching the Chumash, I found that, according to archeologists,[45] the area was originally settled 13,000 years ago. Again, the 26,000-year cycle appears to be in play. The Chumash Indian homeland lies along the coast of California, between Malibu and Paso Robles, as well as on the Northern Channel Islands. The various tribes, numbering approximately 150, traded amongst themselves and the indigenous population. This trade was made possible in part by the seagoing plank canoe or tomol. The currency used in these trades was money made from shells.

I also found that some of the dress of the Chumash resembled that of the Hawaiians. It seems that the Chumash wore grass skirts. These grass skirts or aprons were fashioned from twined cords of cottonwood bark held together with nettles cordage. The grass skirt was sometimes worn alone or in combination with a skirt that was made from cottonwood inner bark ribbons twined together with nettles cordage.

---

43 *The Rainbow Bridge* by Audrey Wood and Robert Florczak (Illustrator), published by Voyager Books; Reprint edition (April 3, 2000), ISBN 015202106X.

44 Lemuria, or Mu, is believed to be an ancient civilization that predates all known or mythological societies. Lemuria is reported to have been inhabited by highly evolved, very Spiritual beings and is believed to have been located in the Southern Pacific between South America and Australia.

45 The Santa Barbara Museum of Natural History web site has a wealth of information on the Chumash people. See http://www.sbnature.org/research/anthro/chumash/index.htm.

I was intrigued and tried to determine if travel between Hawaii and California was possible. I then found the following information associated with a Chumash holy site, Point Humqaq, which is considered by the Chumash as the location of the portal where souls of the dead ascend into the heavens.

Theo Radic described his experiences at Point Humqaq, west of Santa Barbara, California in his book *Crazy Devil Sweeping: A Janitor's Reflections on Art and Tao* (Syukhtun Editions), as sacred – and he likened the area to a shrine. Seaman Richard Henry Dana, in *Two Years Before the Mast* (published 1949 by Literary Guild of America), related that winds around Point Humqaq were so fierce that his ship, sailing north to San Francisco, had to sail nearly to Hawaii to circumvent the winds.

I find it very interesting that the Chumash apply sacred status to an area that has produced the atmospherics necessary to facilitate travel to Hawaii.

As final confirmation that this travel was possible, I found a reference by Lahe'ena'e Gay in the Spring/Summer 1996 issue of the *American Indian Ritual Object Repatriation Foundation Newsletter*. An article in that newsletter described a meeting of indigenous elders called the *Festival of Life* that was held in Vienna, Austria in 1995. At this meeting, Native Hawaiian elders met with Grandfather Semu Huaute, an 87-year-old Chumash medicine man and reportedly the last full-blooded Chumash in California. The Hawaiian elders were led by spirit to adopt Grandfather Semu into the ohana or family.

Later that year, while Grandfather Semu was in Hawaii to attend his formal welcoming into his new family, stories were exchanged of red-skinned people who traveled across the seas to Hawaii in planked canoes. Both the Hawaiians and the red-skinned people spoke the same or a similar language. Grandfather Semu had been told similar stories of how his ancestors had traveled to islands in the middle of the sea. Grandfather Semu commented on the need for native peoples to unify and present one voice to the world.

They, the ancestors and the peoples of present day, were and are, <u>one</u>.

These tantalizing clues lead me to believe that the Chumash were part of the original people who left Hawaii and came to America. I have found that the cultures were similar (seafarers, grass skirts, shell money) and that the winds in the area would have been favorable for travel between the two locations.

Additionally, there are references to similar belief systems in Central and South America. The calendar of the Mayan, the 12,500-year old pyramids in Tiahuanaco, Mexico and other examples lead one to believe that the migration of ancient peoples from Asia, through Polynesia and into the Americas, is a distinct possibility.

Chapter 7: The Future

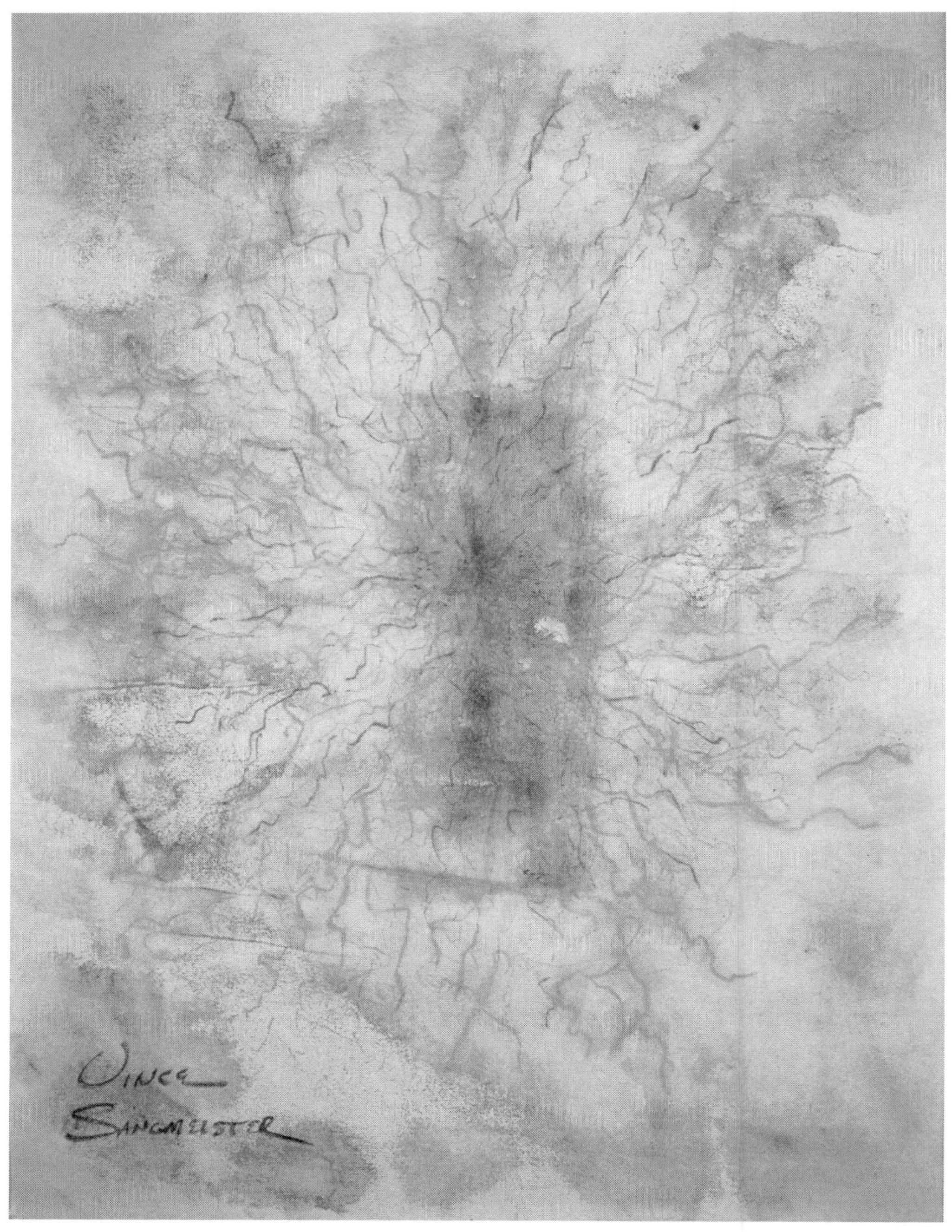

"Drawn to the Doorway"

The paths have connected...we are One entering the doorway!

We are all born with the perfect power to do and be all things. We have the right to do with it whatever we wish...we can go forward and backward in time, walk with the angels, climb the heights and live in paradise. It is everyone's own decision where and what he is.

(Excerpt from *Tales from the Night Rainbow* by Koko Willis and Pali Jae Lee)

The complex lives that we lead can blind us to the beauty and simplicity that surround us. This beauty is God's work. You, I, and everyone else in the world are part of this work. We need to take to time to realize this, see this beauty and connect with all things.

The world is populated by beauty and things that some would describe as ugly. The "ugliness" is often the center of the news we read and the thoughts of the world. The beauty is overlooked and taken for granted. What we do not see and honor, will not be ours to keep.

You can begin to change this pattern by honoring the beauty around you, your environment, your family, the air you breathe, the water you drink, the food you eat. All of these things are gifts from God. As a gift given out of selfless love, your only responsibility is to accept it and say "Thank You!" This simple act of gratitude, even if the air is not perfectly clean or the food is not enough, is honoring these gifts.

The Koran 14.7 says, "...your Lord made it known: If you are grateful, I would certainly give to you more..."

When Morihei Ueshiba O'Sensei spoke on Aikido, he often referred to it as the "Art of Peace." One of the primary focuses of this art is that it begins at home...in you. O'Sensei spoke of first working on yourself...knowing your path and the "contract" that you are here to fulfill. O'Sensei saw that to know peace in the world, you must first know peace inside yourself. Many people try to "fix" the world but fail to realize that they themselves still have areas that need "fixing." As they are One with all that they perceive, they need to work primarily on the only part of the whole that they control: their personal part.

The world can be changed. This is a daunting task that many consider impossible. Start with yourself. If you change yourself for the better, honoring the Divine in all, then...

...the world WILL change!

I hope you have enjoyed following along on this journey. I also hope that you will be journeying out on your own now.

Do your work...you will not be disappointed – I guarantee it! If you do, we will all benefit.

Appendix A: Recommended Reading

The following books are excellent resources on the underlying principles of Oneness.

Children of the Rainbow: The religion, legends and gods of pre-Christian Hawaii

Author:	Leinani Melville
Publisher:	The Theosophical Publishing House
ISBN:	0-8356-0002-5
Description:	Excellent background on Hawaiian spirituality. Out of print and difficult to find; however, a good source is http://www.abebooks.com

Soul Retrieval: Mending the Fragmented Self

Author:	Sandra Ingerman
Publisher:	Harper Collins
ISBN:	0-06-250406-1
Description:	Describes the basic understanding of illness from the Shamanistic perspective of soul loss.

The Laws of Spirit: A Tale of Transformation

Author:	Dan Millman
Publisher:	HJ Kramer
ISBN:	0-915811-93-6
Description:	Explanation of key ideals to live by. Although not directly stated, it is based on Hawaiian spiritual beliefs.

Sacred Journey of the Peaceful Warrior

Author:	Dan Millman
Publisher:	HJ Kramer
ISBN:	0-915811-34-0
Description:	A fictional account of Dan's spiritual growth based on fact. Contains a vast amount of Hawaiian spirituality, including detailed explanations of the "Three Selves."

Spiritwalker: Messages from the Future

Author:	Hank Wesselman, Ph.D.
Publisher:	Bantam
ISBN:	0-553-37837-6
Description:	Detailed information on Kahuna practices as experienced during Dr. Wesselman's own Shamanic journeys into the future. First book in a series.

Medicinemaker: Mystic Encounters on the Shaman's Path

Author:	Hank Wesselman, Ph.D.
Publisher:	Bantam
ISBN:	0-553-37932-1
Description:	Detailed information on Kahuna practices as experienced during Dr. Wesselman's own Shamanic journeys into the future. Second book in a series.

VisionSeeker: Shared Wisdom from the Place of Refuge

Author:	Hank Wesselman, Ph.D.
Publisher:	Hay House
ISBN:	1-56170-753-8
Description:	Detailed information on Kahuna practices as experienced during Dr. Wesselman's own Shamanic journeys into the future. Third book in a series.

The Journey to the Sacred Garden: A Guide to Traveling in the spiritual Realms

Author:	Hank Wesselman, Ph.D.
Publisher:	Hay House
ISBN:	1-4019-0111-5
Description:	A guidebook to Shamanic journeying. A CD of drumming and rattling is included.

The Heart of Huna

Author:	Laura Kealoha Yardley
Publisher:	Advanced Neuro Dynamics
ISBN:	0-9623272-1-2
Description:	Direct telling of Hawaiian spiritual beliefs from a Hawaiian Kaula or light carrier.

Tales from the Night Rainbow

Author:	Koko Willis and Pali Jae Lee
Publisher:	Night Rainbow Publishing Company
ISBN:	0-9628030-0-6
Description:	Tales from ancient Molokai. Contains many ancient references potentially to the ARCH® energies.

The Rainbow Bridge

Author:	Audrey Wood
Publisher:	Voyager Books Harcourt, Inc.
ISBN:	0-15-265475-5
Description:	Re-telling of the creation story of the Chumash Indians of Central California.

Appendix B: Recommended Training

I recommend the following training to further your understanding of Ancient Rainbow Conscious Healing, Shamanism, Hawaiian spirituality and Oneness.

Seminar Series for Ancient Rainbow Conscious Healing
(See website for complete listing of seminars, dates and locations.)

Teacher:	Laurie Keako'a' Grant (or one of the instructors certified by Laurie to teach the first course in the series, the Ancient Rainbow Conscious Healing seminar.)
Length:	Normally 3 days.
Website:	http://www.archhealing.com

Shamanism Training
Spiritwalker: Core Shamanism
Medicinemaker: Shamanic Healing
The Mystical Nature of the Self
Ancestral Spirits
Visionseeker Retreats:
- *Visionseeker Level 1: Shamanism and the modern mystical movement*
- *Visionseeker Level 2: Spirit Medicine*
- *Visionseeker Level 3: Cosmology*

Various conferences and tours (See website for details)

Teacher:	Hank Wesselman
Length:	1 to 7 days
Website:	http://www.sharedwisdom.com

Basic Workshop in Core Shamanism
Advanced Weekend Workshops in Core Shamanism
Advanced Five-Day and Longer Training Courses in Core Shamanism
Special Advanced Five-Day Training Course

Teacher:	The Foundation for Shamanic Studies
Length:	2 to 5 days
Website:	http://www.Shamanism.org

Shamanism Training (continued)

Medicine for the Earth Gatherings:

Five-Day Medicine for the Earth Gathering

Weekend Medicine for the Earth Gatherings

Medicine for the Earth Teacher Training

Reconnecting with Nature: A Shamanic Approach

Advanced Healing

The Way of the Shaman

Five-Day Soul Retrieval Training

Various conferences and tours (See website for details)

Teacher: Sandra Ingerman
Length: 1 to 5 days
Websites:
http://www.Shamanicvisions.com/ingerman.html
or
http://www.medicinefortheearth.com

Oneness Healing Seminar

Teacher: Mark Perkins
Length: 1 to 5 days
Websites: http://www.Onenessjourneys.com

Conferences

Various conferences and tours (See website for details)

Teacher: Gregg Braden
Length: Varied
Website: http://www.greggbraden.net

Spirit-based Conferences (See website for details)

Teacher: The Prophets Conference
Length: Varies
Website: http://www.greatmystery.org

Appendix C: Notes about the Artwork

An introduction from the artist:

"Mark Perkins and I had initially agreed that I would read a draft copy of his book, **My Journey Back to Oneness**, and work from the imagery it gave me to create artwork to serve as "chapter covers" and a book cover. Honestly, I failed miserably in my initial attempts to visualize or interpret the individual chapters. I've never been able to create a painting based on someone else's vision of what that painting should look or feel like. Frustrated beyond belief and with a deadline staring me in the face, I contacted Mark and asked permission to go on a different path. Knowing that I always paint well to music, I requested that Mark make a CD of music that is influential in Mark's work or important in his life. My hope was that perhaps by listening to Mark's musical selections[46] as well as reading the book, I would be able to get a "feel" for the spirit of each chapter and the book as a whole. And then my goal was to depict the musical influence on me instead of painting a visualization of the words. Mark gave me carte blanche to produce whatever I wanted.

"One very rainy Wednesday, I was listening to Mark's CDs when I had what can only be described as an epiphany or revelation. I started to draw and paint as if possessed. As one song ended and another began I put aside the previous piece and started a new one. At one point, I had perhaps forty or fifty sheets strewn about the floor. All were very different.

"I always note what song or album is playing during each painting session. When I resume a certain painting, I'm able to refer to my notes, put on the same music and somehow drift back into the same frame of mind I was in prior to putting the painting aside. What you are about to read are the notes I scribbled everywhere on little scraps of paper. They reference my frame of mind, the music, what the painting is asking for, a final summation or random thoughts that pop into my head as I progress through each piece. This is essentially a diary of these works.

---

46 *Note from Mark:* The music that I sent Vince was a smattering of tunes that seemed to fit the thoughts, feelings and emotions that I wanted the art to express. Artists included Andreas Wollenveider, Pat Metheny, Lyle Mays, Santana, Dave Mathews Band, Hank Wesselman, Hemi-Sync® from the Monroe Institute, Michael Harner, Stephen Mc Donnell and One Heart.

"One quick but vitally important note...My paintings are titled based on the premise that I don't wish to influence what viewers *should* be seeing. I feel what the viewers experience is not for me to predetermine. I much prefer to delegate that responsibility to each individual viewer who will be influenced by his or her respective experiences. I go to great lengths to hide my own experience in creating a work - and I strive to challenge viewers to discover their own revelations. The most flattering compliment to me as an artist, is if you find a connection to any of my works. If you do, I ask that you contact Mark and arrange to see the originals. Until then, enjoy the works (and their notes!) made especially for this book."

– Vince Sangmeister, Bryn Mawr, PA

Heaven, Earth and Between... (Cover oil painting) Never used 300lb water color paper before... I've never used any of these materials (watercolor paper and crayons) before...only oils and canvas... Mark and I talked about recurrent groups or numbers he has noticed... evidently the number three pops up over and over... The Trinity... three primary colors... heaven, hell and earth... earth, wind and fire... I want major blocks of laminated canvas and long colorful drips to represent "heaven" or the sun... lowest blocks (the) earth... us and nature... how to define the in-between part though?? ... this might work... instead of defining the center specifically I used the three primary colors of blue, red and yellow... every color in creation emanates from these three... the basis for all color interpretation... (the painting) needs something iconographic to really tie it to the spirit of the book, but nothing specific to any particular belief system... generic iconography??? ... I really like the way this moves from the top to the bottom... underpainting works in daylight really well... very dark by artificial light... paint at night look at the result during the day in the sunlight... so it goes... this is screaming for me to add other elements... groups of three... groups of three... groups of three... 3, 3, 3, 3, 3,3,3,3... bought three lengths of metal wire, 24k gold, sterling silver and copper wire... the three metals, gold for heaven, copper for earth and silver for all the in-between... braided lengths of wire into different braid patterns and cut pieces off... pierced the painting and tied them together on the backside... took care to tie them off neatly... (I) hate when things look unfinished or like an afterthought... bottom form needs 3 separate entities but how??? ... "glued" down some "stones" I made by mixing paint, medium and sand... sort of a rusty, red color... unitized the stones to the surface by tying wire around them and piercing the paper... don't want (the) bindings to be nice and straight rather more random in nature... like nature, actually... few things in nature are perfectly symmetrical... I just fiddled with those binding wires for over 5 hours... put two braids of wire across the "sun" shape at the top on an angle... removed one since it wants to actually pierce the heavy yellow paint... one above the surface, one actually piercing the paint as if wounding or stabbing or becoming “one” with the yellow form... I need some coffee badly... again, with Starbucks being closed... they should call ahead and give me last call... found a twig on my way back from the store and removed the piercing... replaced it with the twig... pulled small pieces of the rubbery paint up over the twig in spots to grip it or envelope it to sort of nurture it... like this... very cool texture here... placed long wires across the right side canvas form, one over the top the other beneath it but looked too much like a crucifix... needs to be more suggestive in nature and not so blatant... veryyyyyyyy cool... put two outer, smaller braids at the ends of what used to be the cross member that sort of float by themselves but tie together the long canvas piece from a distance... this is neat... this is most certainly NOT what Mark had envisioned... omg, what if it doesn't work??? ... then what??? ... sent off the second package... now to sweat... hope they like my weirdness... emailed Mark telling him it was on its way... DONE!

Swift to Associate... (watercolor) Sunday night... I gotta get cable... no I don't... zilch but PBS on TV... a show on psychology... white noise and music... very neat... this music is interesting... too funny, (the music) fits the show actually. What is this guy babbling about??? (The) forms sort of flow into each other... like an attractive sort of energy between each successive shape... kind of puffy though... like clouds. (I) need to define them a bit more... used black... (The) music is sort of round and soft... blues and whites... outlined in black/white... I like this one... it's kind of peaceful to look at... sort of serene... tis neat... oh cool... PBS psychology show used the term "swift to associate" ... how cool... it fits... thanks PBS and viewers like you for naming my painting... send this one, too...

CD-1.Cut-1... (watercolor) CD1/Song1... emailed Mark about my idea to try this based on this song. Described in the email what the music made me "see" ... It's like a battle being engaged... good vs. evil, nature vs. the unnatural, black vs. white... a far-off challenge... (an) impending storm threatening and stabbing at the coast or beach... this music has a very Caribbean feel to it... What is this painting asking for... omg... put the painting in the tub... figured since it was about a storm, I'd give it a storm... turned on the shower to pelt the shapes with beads of water... like the spray at a beach... held the painting up so the colors drifted together and blended a bit... no longer definitive edges to the color... back in the tub... in the middle... aimed the shower above it so the water runs down the S-shaped ridges on the bottom of the tub... the thingees put there so I don't slip... this is coolllllllllllllllllll... how do you explain to someone that your shower was an integral part of the process? Too funny... the water ran down the grooves in the tub and UNDER the paper and pulled some paint along with it... (At) the end of the song the victor is obvious... good wins... nature wins... the storm did no damage... added salt to the wet paper for texture... needs a lot more texture... salted paper... hmmm... a new snack option?? Send this.

Metropolitan Vortices...(watercolor) It's trying to capture the action of the city at night... walls behind... buildings so to speak... neat color here... neat effect too... in front of the walls (the marks) are very active... like specters... like the wind whipping up a tiny tornado of leaves and debris on the street... pretty cool piece... very subtle but strong composition, I think...subdued colors make it work more nicely... wouldn't work in green, for sure... send this too.

Filtered and Refocused... (watercolor) this thing is going NO WHERE... (I'm) gonna soak it (and) see what happens... this is veryyyyyy cool. (The paint) bled through (and I) really like the effect on the reverse side... great... now I have to start worrying if the bleed is better than the front painting... like the paper filtered the paint... divided it up... like coffee filter paper. (The) music is sort of like that... it's thin... (it's) airy and almost imperceptible at times. omg... nine hours so far tinkering... this is cool though... I like it. I need coffee... cat is drinking my watercolor mixtures... idiot cat... Why can't Starbucks be a 24-hour operation... (they) get you hooked then close... This is really neat... it's taken on a linguistic feel... ancient though, runic in nature... like some sort of symbolic language... love languages... send this one.

Lucid Dream II... (watercolor) WOWWWWWWWWW... this (music) is wild... really electric... very energetic and active... razor sharp. My god, I'm exhausted... see ya' in the mornin'... when am I gonna be able to sleep again?? ... I'm tired... man... 2 whole hours sleep... woooo hoooo... very cool dream though. (This) happened when I did Lucid Dream... each image flashed through my mind like a strobe... veryyyyyyy active and alive... a darkness there though... kind of ominous and threatening the whole... like an impending aggression of some sort... coming from somewhere not so nice... red... and more black... a lot more black... then white... don't want gray to evolve though... got away with it and no mud... Now this is a reallyyyyyyyyy interesting painting... a bit disturbing but very aggressive... definitely send this...

Drawn To The Doorway... (watercolor) 2nd song on the very first CD... cool stuff, Mark... how many days of rain in a row will we get??? Enough already... very, very energetic marks, all eminating from a common center... very bright, fiery color... no shapes just marks... like sparks or lightning sprites... I'm thirsty... it stopped raining before I headed out of the gallery... whew... this painting needs something really badly... no cohesion to it at all... all over the place... needs something to center it badly... more rain... should put the painting out in the rainstorm... cool idea... drew very heavily onto a second sheet in jet black... really soaked the black shape in the center of the second sheet and liquefied the watercolor stick to make it nice and runny... few sprays on the original but not as wet as the black shape... hopefully the original will draw the water and the paint from the second piece... laminated the two together face to face to transfer the black image to the original... need a roller to smoosh them together... this experiment is gonna be a disaster... this is soooooo cool... pulled the two sheets apart... black image transferred but sort of in a ghostly way and slightly offcenter and askew... excellent... I can't stand symmetry... I like this... my favorite so far... like the energy is being sucked into a phantom doorway... really like the light at the bottom of the door.

Blue Agony Resurrection... (oil painting done prior to the artwork for the book) The title *Blue Agony Resurrection* is a combination of three titles for two paintings. Initially I was working on a very loose piece that simply would not cooperate with me. As such, I started to aggressively scrape the paint from the canvas and in doing so I ripped a hole in it damaging the surface. At the time, it was the only canvas I had access to so I set about fixing it. I began working with that color blue and really loved the way it came together. As the painting neared completion, I was initially going to title it very simply, *Blue*. However, since it was being reworked from scratch on a canvas which was moments before destined for the trash the title became *Blue Resurrection,* marking the re-breathing of life into the canvas itself. A while later during a somewhat depressed moment in my life, I completed the painting but now this particular blue took on an entirely different connotation for me. The marks were still very loose but the color seemed to connote something a bit more introspective and personal. Once I finished it, on the back of the painting, I noticed there was a small space between the words "Blue" and "Resurrection." In a different color I added the word "Agony" to mark that moment in my life when I completed the work. By adding the word "Agony" to the title it allowed me to recall that depressed moment in my life but at the same time to file it away where it belonged...on the back of the canvas. Were it on the front it would still be in view and it would still be in the present...it needed to be in the past and out of sight.

Solitary Man... (watercolor) Awesome music... artist???? (I'm) glad Mark didn't write who each artist was on the CDs... no preconceived notions on what to expect based on the artist... Very cool music but sort of... ummm... word??? ... sort of singular... Reminds me of when I'm feeling lonely or alone, like now... but not in a bad or depressive way... more reflective in nature... definitely a reflective event in my life. A human form but androgynous... and from the back... not so readily identifiable as male or female or even human... but it's a guy. (I) wonder who it is?... Probably a self portrait... (that's) all I need, another mirror... Very cool... I love these marks... sort of an Asian feel to it... sorta... like Japanese brush paintings...Very emotive. Wow...this red soooooooo belongs here... awesome red. It (the red color) fits. This painting rocks!!!!! ... send it.

Coeur... (watercolor) French for heart...coeur de leon...heart of the lion right??...listening to a piece of music chosen by Mark Perkins... (It's) a really different piece and sort of drones along. Very constant drumming almost in a ritualistic way... like a heartbeat... The shapes want to be of human form not so much of the outer body but more internal in a biological way. More black... and white over the top of all the kidney shapes... heart shapes. (I'm) gonna let it sit for awhile and just stare at it...where are my smokes?? ... (it will) tell me where it wants to go... at least I hope so... I like this or where it's headed... the music came through pretty well I think... nice and round... very yellow and blue... include this one.

Fractured Self... (watercolor) Interesting music today... heard most of it before but (it) takes on a different relevance depending on (my) mood... (I) want this to be an exploded view of the psyche, id or ego... interesting choice of color... can't stand green... never have liked it... here... though. it works very well... fractured pieces of human spirit here... human form is on the right but barely recognizable as such anymore... (the) vast majority of the shapes and forms are sharp and jagged or angular... nothing smooth here... nothing graceful or round... (the) music is the same way going in 20 different directions at the same time... the undertones going one way, (the) lead, rhythm and percussion all spiraling out of control...sort of like jazz... cool piece, though... will change my mind on this one regarding green... still don't like it, though... this is a pretty neat piece... very introspective... the forms allow me to move in and out pretty easily... send this one.

Active... (watercolor) (I) found that you can make a puddle of the dry (water color) material then wet my fingers and finger paint... this is fun... I feel like a kid and I hated being a kid...music is like that... sort of happy-go-lucky but without the bad parts... very bright... red and blue on white paper... I hope no one thinks this is in a patriotic vein... be careful of using red, white and blue predominately... too many will be wrongfully quick to associate the piece with Americanism... this is pretty cool but it's really missing something to tie all these marks together... drew a heavy white strip across the top... dripped water through the swath to let it wash down over the marks... this definitely works... some of the white transferred to the paper slightly but the water pulled the color of the marks it hit downward... pushes all the marks back... pretty cool here - instead of putting VINCE on the piece, I put my five fingerprints on the top right and trailed them to the left... neat... five letters in VINCE, five fingerprints... this is nice and airy... sort of like art-lite... don't have to think too much... send.

The Attempt (to Heal)... (watercolor) Neat stuff on this song... and the previous 3 or 4... they all fit together. (It's) like the center shape is trying to elicit help from the outside... using the advice or energy from outside to heal itself... needs a lot of help... but can't do it on its own... more color... more help... one side open or missing... it's incomplete... has to be missing... it's incomplete and is trying to repair the broken side... cool piece... I like it... gonna send.

Centered White... (watercolor) I do NOT like where this painting is headed... (The) music is really cool but I'm missing something important in the translation... just NOT getting it... This needs to be opened up in the center with a thin wash of white for some reason... what this needs is a doctor of paintology... I am NOT sending this out to Colorado... no way. omg (Oh my god)... I hate this thing... it's complete mud... all the colors are mud... overworked... quit while (I'm) ahead. yuck... I've picked a dozen to work on... this is gonna be number 13... it deserves that number for sure... against better judgment send it... let them decide... credibility in serious jeopardy with this uglyfest... is that a word???

Interstice II... (watercolor) Gonna try to do the buildings across the street from the gallery... another gray day... raining off and on... buildings are good with this music... the same sort of linear structure in both... this is pretty cool... sort of block in subtle color... build it outward like the building itself... washed over the surface slightly to pull the lower color through a bit more in spots... small white marks like windows or lights or lives in a building... my favorite piece... send this for sure.

Appendix D: Book Creators and their Contact Information

Mark Perkins, author

Mark has worn many hats in his life and traveled many places, with all those experiences playing significant roles in his current spirituality and healing work. He approached these subjects with a logical mind, a scientific eye and a wide-open heart. He constantly encourages others to embark on spiritual journeys, so that they may "do the work" and rejoin themselves with the Divine Source Energy...a philosophy that he even tries to integrate into the "corporate world" whenever possible. He currently conducts healing seminars and individual sessions in Boulder, CO where he lives with his wife and their two children. Please feel free to reach out to Mark by phone at 303-530-3068, via his website (www.onenessjourneys.com) and/or e-mail (mark@onenessjourneys.com).

Vince Sangmeister, artist

Vince is mostly a self-taught painter who works predominately with oils. Currently, his paintings are abstract, large in format, heavily layered and highly textured with elements recurring in nature like sand, twigs and stones. Armed with coffee and music, "night owl" Vince spends many a night in his Bryn Mawr, PA studio, capturing his kinetic creations on canvas in the hopes of pulling viewers into the work and creating a mirror onto themselves. His paintings hang in private collections (nationally and internationally) as well as in the 3rd Street Gallery in Philadelphia, PA. Vince donates a portion of his proceeds to charities that benefit Juvenile Diabetes and Multiple Sclerosis. You can view Vince's works on the gallery website (www.3rdstreetgallery.com) or contact him directly at the gallery (215-625-0993) or via e-mail (vncntsng@aol.com).

Rose Boden, photographer

Rose is an artist that works in different mediums. Weekdays you can find her up on a ladder creating cozy living spaces as she paints interiors - and many weekends you can find her pursuing her other passion: photography. Her photographic credits include capturing life's celebrations (weddings, bar mitzvahs and birthdays) and nature's outdoor beauty. She lives on a beautiful mountain property in Woodland Park, Colorado with her partner, their three children and a bunch of friendly creatures, large and small. Please feel free to contact her at stockpaint2@aol.com.

ISBN 141200903-0

9 781412 009034